Slim Eating Guide

Simple Everyday Cooking for Natural Weight Loss

Table of Contents

Skinny Breakfast Egg Scramble

Green Baked Avocado

Baked Egg Muffins

Pancakes with Berry Topping

Almond Butter Crunch Granola Bar

Superfood Granola Bowl

Skinny Raisin Rugalach

Double Chocolate Chip Scone

Very Berry Fruit Cereal

Spicy Kale with Poached Eggs

Morning Mellow Melon

Bright & Early Orange Whirl

Hearty Apple Almond Salad

Sweet Citrus Salad with Coconut Cream

Superfood Breakfast Brownies

Slim 'n' Trim Vegetarian Dishes

Low-Carb Spicy Kale Quiche

Eggplant with Pesto Topping

Spicy Zucchini Eggplant Dine

Lettuce Nut Salad

Eggplant with Red Sauce

Sweet Potatoes Roast

Pepper Quiche

"Green Bean" Casserole

Mushroom Masala

Easy Matzo Ball Soup

Butternut Squash Soup

Mexican Tomato Soup

Creamy "Cheesy" Broccoli Soup

Pita Bites

Simple Gazpacho + Tortilla Chips

Grain-Free Tortillas

Veggie Burger

Soft Burger Buns

Skinny Egg Salad Sandwich

Sandwich Bread

Kelp Noodle Salad

Zucchini Salad with Sundried Tomato Sauce

Quick Raw Avocado Slaw

Vegetarian Texas Chili

Skinny Caesar Salad

Spiced Walnut Autumn Salad

Pecan Apricot Spinach Salad

Southern Style Egg Salad

Pesto Tomato Caprese

Cashew Crunch Kelp Noodle Salad

Dill Stuffed Tomatoes

Squash Blossom Stuffers

Indian Egg Fried Rice

Skinny Munchies

Spicy Chicken Wraps

Fruit Salad

Tahini with Fruit Topping

Skinny Frozen Coconut

Black Pepper & Kale Chips

Nuts & Raisin Bars

Tart Cherry Energy Bar

Simple Almond Apricot Balls

Simple Spiced Honey Nuts

Zucchini Fries

Skinny Jalapeño Lime Hot Wings

Pancetta Wrapped Shrimp Snacks

Sundried Tomato Cashew Hummus with Carrots

Chocolate Hazelnut Spread with Apples

Chocolate Chia Pudding

Holy Loaded Guacamole

Bacon Quesadilla

Baked Sweet Plantains

Ants On A Log

Chocolate Banana Bites

Piña Colada Smoothie

Jalapeño Bacon Bites

Green Deviled Eggs 'N Ham

Cocoa Cream Bun

Chicken Tenders

Homemade Applesauce

Strawberry Banana Shake

Mango Ginger Apple Salad

Tuna Spread

Slim Mocha Brownie Bites

Sea-riously Good Skinny Recipes

New England Clam Chowder

Calamari with Ginger Sauce

Thai Steamed Mussels

Chinese Mustard Baked Salmon

Skinny Baked Tilapia Filets

Fresh Sashimi Bento Bowl

Fresh Clams with Cocktail Sauce

Asian Shrimp Lettuce Wraps

Smoked Salmon Avocado Salad

Tuna Tartar with Avocado and Mango

City Clam Chowder

Salmon Tartar Stack

Garlic and White Wine Steamed Mussels

Shrimp Stuffed Squid

Lobster Newburg

Seafood Paella

Skinny Tuna Tartar Crêpes

Smoked Salmon Eggs Benedict

Seared Tuna Salad

Tilapia Ceviche

Oyster Po' Boy

Long Rolls

Tuna Sandwich

Sandwich Bread

Healthy Shrimp Taco

Grain-Free Tortillas

Coconut Shrimp

Clams Casino

Crispy Soft Shell Crab With Garlic Lemon Aioli

Almond Crusted Pan Seared Scallops

Basque Style Cod Fish Stew

Delicious Lobster Bisque

Red Snapper Soup

Simple Sweet & Savory Bread Recipes

Cheesy Jalapeño "Cornbread"

Pure Pumpkin Bread

Gluten-Free Poppy Seed Pretzel

Blueberry Scones

Cinnamon Raisin Bread

Skinny Classic Bagels

Candied Banana Bread

Onion Crumpets

Rosemary Basil Scones

Fennel Breakfast Biscuits

Kefir Sourdough Rolls

Everything Bagels

Skinny Egg Bread

Cocoa Gingerbread

Apple Bread

Plain Pita

All-Purpose Pizza Crust

Strawberry Bread

Citrus Curry Spice Bread

Cranberry Pistachio Scones

Sweet Potato Basil Rolls

Low-Carb English Muffins

Indian Naan

Soft Burger Buns

Sandwich Bread

Grain-Free Tortillas

Double Chocolate Chip Scone

Pretzel Sticks

Sweet Banana Shortbreads

Lemon Lavender Scones

Indulgent Baked Treats

Strawberry Toaster Pastry

Cocoa Zucchini Muffin

Vanilla Bean Shortbread Cookies

Cranberry Pistachio Biscotti

Skinny Cherry Pie

Berry Cobbler

Vanilla Peach Cake

Lemon Bundt Cake

Chocolate Zucchini Cake

Ginger Spice Cookies

Orange Cranberry Muffins

Milano Cookie Sandwiches

Cocoa Spice Pinwheel Cookies

Skinny Key Lime Coconut Bars

Coconut Baked Donut

Soft Pumpkin Cookies

Asian Orange Muffins

Coconut Crisps

Pecan Chess Pies

Mixed Berry Trifle

Sugar Cookies

Apple Dump Muffins

Fruit And Nut Cake

Honey Nut Bun

Orange Anzac Biscuits

Sweet Cherry Fig Newtons

Pineapple Upside Down Cake

Simple Chinese Moon Cakes

Walnut Raisin Cookies

Apple Upside Down Cakes

Guilt Free Desserts

Skinny Apple Crumble

Creamy Pumpkin Cheesecake

Gingerbread Cookies

Basic Banana Bread

Scrumptious Cinnamon Buns

Yummy Strawberry Rhubarb Pie

Sweet Raisin Pecan Cake

Slim Cranberry Almond Cookies

Pineapple Coconut Cake

Mocha Brownie Bites

Cinnamon Raisin Bread

Easy Poppy Seed Muffins

Blackberry Dumplings

Skinny Coconut Baked Donut

Delicious Apple Pastries

Healthy Lemon Coconut Bars

Chocolate Pecan Shortbread Cookies

Red Velvet Bars

Wild Mince Meat Pie

Baked Peaches

Tiramisu

Chocolate Almond Biscotti

Ginger Mango Sherbet

Pineapple Upside Down Cake

Cashew Chocolate Mousse

Sweet Cinnamon Pretzel

Healthy Refrigerator Carrot Cake

Ginger Punch Pudding

Quick Tropical Sorbet

Delicious Weeknight Dinners

Chicken Satay

Skinny Orange Chicken

Cashew Chicken

Spicy Hunan Beef and Broccoli

Meaty Texas Chili

Spicy Meatball Marinara

Highland Sheppard's Pie

Black Pepper Stew

Nuts & Turkey Burgers

Skinny Chicken Bruschetta

Herb Roasted Pork Tenderloin

Ground Beef Stuffed Peppers

Stuffed Cabbage in Tomato Sauce

Slow Cooker Beef Pot Roast

Slow Cooker Beef Burgundy

Spicy Thai Soup

Sweet Potato & Bacon Soup

Parchment Baked Salmon

Chicken Fries with Garlic Aioli

Ethiopian Beef Stew

Veggie Musakhan

Braised Lamb in Tomato Sauce

Garlic Sesame Chicken

Stewed Chicken and Dumplings

Slim 'n' Trim Oven-Fried Chicken

Southern Liver and Onions

Spicy Oregano Cubes

French Country Coq Au Vin

Uptown Clam Chowder

Holiday Baked Ham

Introduction

Have you noticed how many diet foods contain more junk than regular foods? They are filled with artificial sweetener, extra sugar and preservatives. Even if they are low-cal, those skinny frozen dinners probably don't do much for you in terms of nutrition. We have a better solution: delicious homemade meals containing generous amounts of meats and veggies to make you feel full without overloading on carbs. Natural meats and veggies are loaded with good stuff and contain different compounds that can help you achieve your weight-loss goals. Try these easy dinner ideas and you will wonder why you ever bothered with diet foods!

Quick and Healthy Breakfast Ideas

Breakfast Buns

Prep Time: 15 minutes

Cook Time: 20 minutes

Servings: 4

INGREDIENTS

Breakfast Bun

1 cup tapioca flour

1/4 - 1/3 cup coconut flour

1 cage-free egg

1/2 cup warm water

1/4 cup coconut oil

Bacon drippings

2 tablespoons applesauce

1 teaspoon apple cider vinegar

1/2 teaspoon baking soda

1/2 teaspoon ground black pepper

1/4 teaspoon sea salt

Filling

4 cage-free eggs

4 slices nitrate-free bacon

1/2 small bell pepper

1/2 small onion

1/4 teaspoon ground black pepper

1/4 teaspoon sea salt

INSTRUCTIONS

1. Preheat oven to 350 degrees F. Line sheet pan with parchment paper or coat with coconut oil. Heat medium skillet over medium-high heat. Add water to small pot and heat over medium heat.

2. For *Filling*, peel onion, stem, seed and vein pepper, and chop bacon. Add bacon to hot skillet and sauté until bacon is crisp and almost cooked through. Drain off drippings and set aside.

3. Dice onion and pepper and add to bacon. Sauté about 2 minutes, unto bacon is cooked through and veggies are softened. Add eggs and lightly scrambled, just 30 seconds - 1 minute. Remove from heat and set aside.

4. For *Breakfast Bun*, sift together tapioca flour, coconut flour, baking soda, salt and pepper in medium bowl.

5. Whisk egg, applesauce and vinegar in small bowl. Whisk in warm water, coconut oil and bacon drippings.

6. Add egg mixture to flour mixture and mix until well combined. Add 1 tablespoon coconut flour or water at a time if needed to form soft and slightly sticky dough.

7. Divide dough into 4 portions and flatten into round disks. Dust your hand or rolling pin with extra tapioca flour to prevent sticking.

8. Scoop loose egg *Filling* into center of each dough disk and pinch edges of dough together to create round, sealed ball.

9. Place filled buns sealed side down on sheet pan and pat down slightly.

10. Place in oven and bake 20 minutes, or until edges are golden brown and dough is cooked through.

11. Remove from oven and let cool about 5 minutes.

12. Serve warm.

Avocado Club Muffin

Prep Time: 10 minutes

Cook Time: 15 minutes

Servings: 12

INGREDIENTS

1 cup almond flour

2 cage-free eggs

1 avocado

4 slices nitrate-free bacon

1 tablespoon sweetener*

1 teaspoon apple cider vinegar

1 teaspoon baking powder

1/4 teaspoon ground white pepper (or black pepper)

INSTRUCTIONS

1. Preheat oven to 350 degrees F. Line muffin pan with paper liners or light coat with coconut oil. Heat medium pan over medium-high heat.

2. Finely chop bacon and add to hot pan. Sauté until crisp and cooked through, about 5 minutes. Set aside.

3. Beat eggs, sweetener and vinegar in medium mixing bowl with hand mixer or whisk until thick and slightly foamy.

4. Slice avocado in half. Scoop flesh of one half into egg mixture. Add bacon and drippings, almond flour, baking powder and black pepper and mix until combined.

5. Dice remaining avocado flesh and fold into batter.

6. Use ice cream scoop or tablespoon to scoop batter into prepared muffin pan.

7. Bake about 15 - 20 minutes, until edges are golden brown and tops are firm.

8. Remove from oven and let cool for 5 minutes.

9. Serve warm. Or cool completely and serve temperature.

NOTE: Bake in square oiled baking pan for 30 - 35 minutes for **Avocado Club Bread**.

stevia, raw honey or agave nectar

Spinach Mushroom Muffins

Prep Time: 10 minutes

Cook Time: 15 minutes

Servings: 12

INGREDIENTS

1 cup almond flour

2 eggs

1 cup fresh spinach

1/2 cup fresh mushrooms

1 tablespoon sweetener*

1 tablespoon apple cider vinegar

1 teaspoon baking soda

1 teaspoon baking powder

1 teaspoon ground white pepper (or black pepper)

1/2 teaspoon ground nutmeg

1/2 teaspoon dried basil

INSTRUCTIONS

1. Preheat oven to 350 degrees F. Line muffin pan with paper liners or lightly coat with coconut oil. Heat medium pan over medium-high heat.

2. Slice mushrooms and add to hot pan. Sauté about 3 minutes, then add spinach. Sauté until water evaporates, mushrooms are cooked through and spinach is wilted. Set aside.

3. Beat eggs, sweetener and vinegar in medium mixing bowl with hand mixer or whisk until thick and frothy.

4. Add sautéed veggies, almond flour, baking soda and powder and spices and mix until combined.

5. Use ice cream scoop or tablespoon to pour batter into prepared muffin pan.

6. Bake 15 - 20 minutes, until edges are golden brown and tops are firm.

7. Remove muffins from oven and let cool about 5 minutes.

8. Serve warm. Or allow to cool complete and serve temperature.

NOTE: Bake in square oiled baking pan for 30 - 35 minutes for **Spinach Mushroom Bread**.

stevia, raw honey or agave nectar

Fennel Breakfast Biscuits

Prep Time: 5 minutes

Cook Time: 15 minutes

Servings: 8

INGREDIENTS

2 1/2 cups fine almond flour (not almond meal)

2 eggs

1/4 cup coconut oil

2 tablespoons fennel seeds

1 teaspoon baking soda

1/2 teaspoon sea salt

1 tablespoon sweetener*

INSTRUCTIONS

1. Preheat oven to 350 degrees F. Line sheet pan with parchment paper.
2. Grind 1 tablespoon fennels seeds in spice grinder or high-speed blender.
3. Combine almond flour, baking soda, salt and ground fennel in medium bowl.
4. Separate egg whites into separate medium bowl, and yolks into small bowl. Beat egg whites to soft peaks with hand mixer or whisk, about 5 minutes.
5. Mix yolks, oil and sweetener into whites. Mix egg mixture into dry ingredients to form soft, solid dough.

6. Roll dough into balls and flatten into 1 inch round biscuits with hands. Place on prepared sheet pan and brush with coconut oil. Sprinkle on whole fennel seeds.
7. Place in oven for 12 - 15 minutes, until golden and firm on top.
8. Remove from oven and serve warm.

NOTE: Oil square baking pan, gently press in dough, use knife or pizza cutter to score in 9 squares, and bake for about 25 minutes for break-away **Fennel BreakfastPan Biscuits**.

stevia, raw honey or agave nectar

Grain-Free Gingerbread

Prep Time: 5 minutes

Cook Time: 20 minutes

Servings: 8

INGREDIENTS

2 cups almond flour

2 tablespoons ground chia seed (or flax meal)

2 eggs

1/2 cup unsweetened applesauce

1/4 cup coconut oil

1/4 cup sweetener*

1 tablespoon baking powder

1 teaspoon baking soda

2 tablespoons ground ginger

1 tablespoon vanilla

1 tablespoon ground cinnamon

1 teaspoon ground black pepper

1/2 teaspoon ground cloves

1/2 teaspoon cardamom (optional)

1 oz fresh ginger juice (optional)

INSTRUCTIONS

1. Preheat oven to 350 degrees F. Coat 2 small loaf pans with coconut oil.

2. In large bowl, beat eggs until light and thickened. Add applesauce, oil, sweetener and ginger juice (optional). Beat well.

3. In medium bowl, blend all dry ingredients well. Slowly stir flour mixture into egg mixture.

4. Pour batter into loaf pans and bake for 20 - 25 minutes, or until toothpick inserted into center comes out clean.

5. Let cool slightly. Insert knife around edges and remove from pan. Serve warm or room temperature.

NOTE: Bake in large oiled loaf pan for 35 - 45 minutes for **Grain-Free Gingerbread Loaf**.

raw honey, agave nectar, grade B maple syrup, molasses

Cranberry Pistachio Scones

Prep Time: 10 minutes

Cook Time: 25 minutes

Servings: 8

INGREDIENTS

2 cups almond flour

1/3 cup arrowroot flour

1 egg

1/4 cup organic coconut oil

2 tablespoons liquid sweetener*

2 teaspoons baking powder

1/2 teaspoon vanilla

1/2 teaspoon sea salt

1/4 cup pistachio nuts

1/4 cup dried cranberries

INSTRUCTIONS

1. Preheat oven to 350 degrees F. Line sheet pan with parchment or coat with coconut oil.
2. Whisk together flours, baking powder, salt and vanilla in large mixing bowl.
3. In small mixing bowl, combine egg, oil and sweetener with hand mixer or whisk. Beat briskly while slowly pouring in coconut oil.
4. Add egg mixture to flour blend and mix until well combined.

5. Fold in cranberries and pistachios until incorporated. Form dough into ball and place on sheet pan . Pat down to flatten to about 1/2 inch thick circle.
6. Cut into eight wedges with pizza cutter or sharp knife. Arrange at least 1 inch apart on sheet pan and bake for 20 - 25 minutes , or until edges are golden brown.
7. Remove and cool. Serve room temperature.

fresh squeezed orange juice, raw honey, agave nectar or grade B maple syrup

Sage Sausage Buns

Prep Time: 10 minutes

Cook Time: 15 minutes

Servings: 8

INGREDIENTS

8 oz uncooked natural sage sausage

3/4 cup coconut flour

4 eggs

1/4 cup unsweetened applesauce

1/4 almond milk

1 teaspoon baking powder

2 tablespoons ground sage

1 tablespoon fresh basil

1 teaspoon ground white pepper (or black pepper)

1/2 teaspoon salt

INSTRUCTIONS

1. Preheat oven to 350 degrees F. Coat muffin pan with coconut oil. Heat medium skillet over medium heat.

2. Brown sausage in skillet for about 5 minutes, until half way cooked. Set aside and reserve leftover oil.

3. While sausage browns, separate eggs. In large bowl, whisk egg whites to soft peaks with hand mixer or whisk. Add yolks, applesauce and almond milk. Mix until combined.

4. Mince basil. Sift flour, baking soda and salt into egg mixture. Add pepper, sage and basil. Stir to combine.

5. Distribute par-cooked sausage evenly into each muffin pan cup. Use ice cream scoop or spoon to scoop batter on top of sausage. Fill each cup no more than 3/4 full.

6. Baste with sausage dripping before placing in oven. Bake 15 - 20 minutes, or until tops are golden brown and firm to the touch.

7. Turn out buns onto plate. Serve warm or room temperature.

NOTE: Bake in oiled square baking pan for 30 - 40 minutes for **Sage Sausage Bread**.

Chicken Breakfast Patties

Prep Time: 5 minutes

Cook Time: 10 minutes

Servings: 2

INGREDIENTS

8 oz chicken

1 egg

1/4 cup coconut flour

1/2 sweet onion

1 tablespoon apple cider vinegar

1 teaspoon ground black pepper

1 teaspoon sea salt

1 teaspoon paprika

1 teaspoon ground sage

1 teaspoon dried thyme

1 teaspoon fennel seed (optional)

1/2 teaspoon nutmeg (optional)

1 tablespoon water

Coconut oil (for cooking)

INSTRUCTIONS

1. Heat medium skillet over medium heat and lightly coat with
   coconut oil.

2. Grind chicken meat and peeled 1/2 onion to medium grind in food processor, bullet blender, or meat grinder. Or grind onion alone and add to pre-ground chicken in medium bowl.

3. Add apple cider vinegar, spices and 1 tablespoon coconut flour to ground chicken and onion. Mix well until combined. Form into 2 large or 4 small patties and place on plate.

4. Beat egg with water and pour egg wash over patties. Gently flip patties to get them evenly covered with egg wash. Take coconut flour and sprinkle over both sides of egg washed patties. Pat coconut flour gently into patties.

5. Place coated patties into hot oiled skillet and cook about 3 - 4 minutes, until golden brown and crisp. Flip and cook another 3 - 4 minutes, or until done.

6. Remove cooked patties from pan and drain on paper towel. Serve hot.

Crunchy Grain-Free Granola

Prep Time: 5 minutes

Cook Time: 20 minutes

Servings: 4

INGREDIENTS

1 cup almond flour

1/4 cup ground chia seed (or flax seed meal)

1 tablespoon vanilla

1 teaspoon ground nutmeg

1 teaspoon ground cinnamon

1/2 cup raw agave nectar (or 1/2 cup raw honey + 1 tablespoon water)

1 cup flaked coconut

1 cup sliced almonds

1/2 cup dried figs

1/2 cup dried dates

1/2 cup pecans

1/2 cup pumpkin seeds

1/2 cup dried apricots

1/2 cup coconut oil, melted

INSTRUCTIONS

1. Preheat oven to 350 degrees F. Lightly coat cookie sheet with coconut oil.

2. Stem figs and pit dates. Chop figs, dates, pecans and apricots. Add to medium bowl, along with all other ingredients. Mix to combine, then spread evenly over sheet pan with spatula.

3. Bake in preheated oven for about 10 minutes. Then carefully remove and use spatula to turn over par-baked granola. Bake for additional 8 - 10 minutes. Check periodically to ensure nuts do not over-toast.

4. Remove from oven and let cool and firm. Serve cool.

Ham, Egg & Veggie Breakfast Burrito

Prep Time: 10 minutes

Cook Time: 10 minutes

Servings: 2

INGREDIENTS

Tortillas:

2 tablespoons coconut flour

2 tablespoons almond flour

2 teaspoons ground flax seed

2 eggs

2 tablespoons melted coconut oil

1/4 teaspoon baking powder

1/4 - 1/2 cup water

Coconut oil (for cooking)

Filling:

6 oz natural pre-cooked ham

6 eggs

1 bell pepper

1/2 red onion

1 avocado

4 oz organic salsa

Pinch sea salt

Pinch ground black pepper

INSTRUCTIONS

1. Heat large pan over medium-high heat and coat with 2 tablespoons of coconut oil. Heat second skillet over medium heat and lightly coat with coconut oil.

2. For *Tortillas*, blend coconut flour, almond flour, flax meal and baking powder in medium bowl. In separate bowl, whisk together 2 eggs, 2 tablespoons coconut oil and 1/4 cup water.

3. Slowly whisk dry blend into wet mixture. Whisk as you pour to avoid clumps. Continue to whisk and slowly add just enough water to make thin but hearty batter.

4. Once coconut oil is hot, use ladle or dry measure cup to pour half of batter into large pan. Tilt pan in circular motion as you pour so batter spreads thinly. Cook batter for about 2 minutes or until tortilla is slightly golden and firm.

5. While *Tortillas* cook, seed and stem pepper and peel onion. Chop ham, pepper and onion. Add to second skillet and sauté for about 2 minutes.

6. Flip tortilla and cook for 2 more minutes. Remove when toasted and cooked through. Place on paper towel or parchment. Add remaining batter to large pan, repeating tilting process to create thin tortilla.

7. While second tortilla cooks , beat 6 eggs in medium bowl and pour over veggies and ham. Salt and pepper to taste. Scramble until desired firmness.

8. Fill both tortillas down center each with half of ham scramble. Slice avocado in half, pit, then scoop out flesh onto each burrito.

9. Roll up tortillas and plate fold-side down. Dollop with your favorite salsa. Serve warm.

Egg In A Hole

Prep Time: 5 minutes

Cook Time: 15 minutes

Servings: 2

INGREDIENTS

Pancakes:

1 3/4 cups almond meal

3/4 cup almond milk

2 eggs

1 teaspoon baking powder

1 teaspoon vanilla

Pinch sea salt

Pinch ground black pepper

Agave nectar (optional)

Coconut oil (for cooking)

Filling:

4 eggs

INSTRUCTIONS

1. Heat large skillet with lid over medium heat and lightly coat with coconut oil.
2. Whisk together 2 eggs, almond milk and vanilla in medium bowl. Whisk in almond flour, baking powder and salt until smooth.

3. Use ladle or dry measure cup to pour 1/3 of batter onto hot oiled skillet in a circle with a hole large enough for one egg. Fit up to 2 pancakes comfortably, so they do not touch as they spread.

4. Crack one egg into each space within pancake. Cover with lid and cook until sides of pancakes are firm and batter bubbles up a bit. About 3 - 4 minutes.

5. Remove lid and gently flip pancakes with spatula, careful to keep yolks intact. Cook uncovered for about 3 minutes, or until pancakes are cooked through.

6. Repeat with remaining batter. Re-oil pan if necessary. Pancakes will be slightly delicate, so flip and plate with care.

7. Sprinkle egg with salt and pepper to taste. Drizzle with agave nectar (optional). Serve warm.

Cowboy Breakfast Skillet

Prep Time: 5 minutes

Cook Time: 15 minutes

Servings: 2

INGREDIENTS

6 eggs

8 oz ground pork sausage

1 medium sweet potato

1 bell pepper

1 small red onion

Ground black pepper, to taste

Paprika, to taste

sea salt, to taste

Pinch of cinnamon (optional)

INSTRUCTIONS

1. Bring medium pot to boil with lightly salted water. Leave enough room in pot for sweet potato. Heat large skillet over medium-high heat.

2. Peel and dice sweet potato. Add to boiling water for 5 minutes.

3. Add sausage to hot skillet. Brown sausage for 5 minutes, stirring occasionally with wooden spatula.

4. While potatoes and sausage cook, seed and vein bell pepper and peel onion, then dice.

5. Beat eggs with spices in medium bowl with hand mixer or whisk.

6. Once browned, add pepper and onion to sausage. Sauté about 2 minutes, until vegetables are tender and a bit caramelized.

7. Drain sweet potatoes in colander and add to skillet. Sauté about 1 minute, until any excess liquid is evaporated. Then pour in egg mixture.

8. Scramble eggs with wooden spatula. Reduce skillet to medium heat to cook eggs evenly and avoid browning.

9. Cook and stir eggs until desired firmness. Remove from heat and serve.

Strawberry Banana Shake

Prep Time: 5 minutes*

Cook Time: 0 minutes

Servings: 1

INGREDIENTS

1 banana

1 cup strawberries

1/2 - 1 cup water

Meat of 1/2 fresh coconut (or 1/2 cup unsweetened flaked or shredded coconut)

INSTRUCTIONS

1. *Soak flaked coconut in water for at least 4 hours.
2. Add fresh or soaked flaked coconut and water to high-speed blender. Process on high until smooth, about 1 minute.
3. Strain coconut mixture through nut milk bag or a few layers of cheese cloth. Squeeze out all excess liquid. Reserve coconut milk. Dry excess coconut, process until finely ground, and use as coconut flour.
4. Remove leaves from strawberries and chop. Peel banana.
5. Add coconut milk to blender with fruit and process on high until smooth.
6. Pour into serving glass and serve immediately.

7. Or chill in refrigerator for 20 minutes, blend for a few seconds to incorporate separated liquid, then pour into serving glass and serve chilled.

Highland Scotch Egg

Prep Time: 10 minutes

Cook Time: 25 minutes

Servings: 6

INGREDIENTS

6 eggs

12 oz ground sausage (pork, chicken, etc.)

1 tablespoon dried parsley

2 teaspoons lemon zest

1/4 teaspoon ground nutmeg

1/4 teaspoon dried sage

Pinch sea salt

Pinch ground black pepper

1 egg

1/2 cup almond meal

Coconut oil (for cooking)

Mustard Sauce

1 egg yolk

1/4 cup coconut oil

1/4 cup organic mustard

2 tablespoons sweetener*

INSTRUCTIONS

1. Bring medium pot of lightly salted water to boil.

2. Carefully place eggs in pot with tongs. Boil eggs for about 10 minutes.

3. For *Mustard Sauce*, add yolk, coconut oil, mustard and sweetener to food processor and bullet blender. Process until emulsified, about 2 minutes. Transfer to serving dish and refrigerate about 15 minutes.

4. Heat small pot over medium heat. Add enough coconut oil to cover width of whole egg, about 2 1/2 inches.

5. Drain eggs and cool under cold running water. Once cool, peel off shells and set aside.

6. Add sausage to medium bowl with parsley, lemon zest, nutmeg, sage, salt and pepper. Mix to combine.

7. Wet hands and cover each whole, peeled egg with a layer of seasoned sausage. Work sausage around eggs and pat into even layer.

8. Pour almond meal into shallow dish. Whisk egg in small bowl. Roll sausage covered eggs in beaten egg, then dredge in almond meal.

9. Carefully place 2 eggs into hot oil and fry for 4 to 5 minutes, until browned and heated through. Turn half way through cooking with tongs.

10. Remove eggs with tongs or slotted spoon and place on paper towel to drain. Repeat with remaining eggs.

11. Serve hot with *Mustard Sauce*.

*stevia, raw honey or agave nectar

NOTE: For *Baked Scotch Eggs*, preheat oven to 400 degrees F and bake coated eggs on wire rack over sheet pan for about 15 minutes, until sausage is fully cooked.

Blueberry Morning Drink

Prep time: 5 minutes

INGREDIENTS

1 handful spinach

½ avocado

1 banana

½ cup blueberries

1 tbsp coconut oil

1 tsp cinnamon

1 cup water

INSTRUCTIONS

1. Slice avocado in half and remove the nut. Break the banana into small pieccs.
2. Combine all ingredients except for the spinach into a blender. Blend them until pureed, then add spinach and blend until pureed.
3. Serve or chill and then serve.

Skinny Breakfast Egg Scramble

Prep time: 5 minutes

Cook time: 3-6 minutes

INGREDIENTS

2 cage-free eggs

1 small onion

1 clove garlic

½ red bell pepper

1 tbsp extra virgin olive oil

¼ tsp smoked paprika

¼ tsp ground black pepper

INSTRUCTIONS

1. Finely chop onion, garlic and red bell pepper.
2. Pour extra virgin olive oil into a pan over medium heat.
3. Crack eggs and pour into a small bowl. Combine with onion, garlic and red bell pepper and whisk until mixed together.
4. Pour contents of bowl into pan and add smoked paprika and ground black pepper. Scramble until desired doneness.
5. Serve.

Green Baked Avocado

Prep time: 3 minutes

Cook time: 15-20 minutes

INGREDIENTS

1 avocado

2 cage-free eggs

⅛ tsp ground black pepper

2 tsp chives

INSTRUCTIONS

1. Preheat oven to 425 degrees.
2. Slice the avocado in half and remove the nut. Scoop out enough flesh from the center of each avocado to contain the contents of 1 egg.
3. Crack the eggs and dump them into the middle of each piece of avocado. Place them on a baking sheet and bake for 15-20 minutes.
4. Remove from oven. Season with pepper and chives and serve.

Baked Egg Muffins

Prep time: 5 minutes

Cook time: 15-20 minutes

INGREDIENTS

1 tbsp olive oil

1 tbsp coconut oil

6 cage-free eggs

1 onion

½ yellow bell pepper

½ red bell pepper

¼ tsp ground black pepper

¼ tsp Celtic sea salt

INSTRUCTIONS

1. Preheat oven to 350. Whisk all 6 eggs in a bowl. Chop the onion and bell pepper into small pieces.
2. In a pan, combine olive oil with onion over medium-high heat for 2 minutes. Add peppers and cook another 2 minutes.
3. Remove onion/peppers from heat and let cool a few minutes. Combine them with the eggs. Add the Celtic sea salt and ground black pepper and mix.
4. Coat a muffin pan with the coconut oil. Fill each muffin cup with the egg/pepper/onion mix. Do not fill a muffin cup more than ¾ full.

5. Place the pan in the oven and bake 10-15 minutes, removing the pan from the oven when the tops of the muffins get fluffy and golden brown.

6. Remove the muffins from the pan and serve.

Pancakes with Berry Topping

Prep time: 10 minutes

Cook time: 20-25 minutes

INGREDIENTS

Pancake

½ cup organic almond butter

½ cup organic applesauce

2 cage-free eggs

¼ tsp cinnamon

Fruit dressing

2 stalks rhubarb

2 cups strawberries

¼ cup water

Toppings

whole strawberries

raw, unfiltered honey

INSTRUCTIONS

1. Chop the rhubarb and slice the strawberries. Place water, rhubarb and strawberries in a saucepan and simmer, covered, for 15 minutes.
2. Remove from heat and mash into a paste, then set aside.

3. Mix almond butter, applesauce, cinnamon and eggs in a bowl. Pour a thin layer of this into a frying pan over medium heat. Flip as you would a pancake and cook until thickened, about 1 to 2 minutes on each side. Set this pancake aside, recoat the bottom of the frying pan with another layer of the mixture, and cook this the same way.

4. Place the first pancake on a plate. Spread the fruit mixture over the surface of this pancake. Place the second pancake on top. Cut the breakfast cake across its diameter into 8 slices.

5. When serving a slice, drizzle with honey and top with 2 strawberries.

Almond Butter Crunch Granola Bar

Prep Time: 30 minutes

Servings: 8

INGREDIENTS

1 1/2 cup raw almonds

1 cup crunchy almond butter

1/4 cup flax seed (or chia seed)

1/2 cup dried pitted dates

2/3 cup shredded or flaked coconut

1/3 cup raw pumpkin seeds

1/2 teaspoon ground cinnamon

1/2 teaspoon vanilla

1 teaspoon Celtic sea salt

INSTRUCTIONS

1. Line loaf pan with parchment paper.
2. Add flax or chia to food processor or high-speed blender and process until finely ground, about 1 - 2 minutes.
3. Add 1 cup almonds and process until thick, smooth paste forms, up to 5 minutes.
4. Add dates and process until thick, fairly smooth mixture forms about 1 - 2 minutes. Transfer to medium mixing bowl.
5. Add remaining 1/2 cup almonds, almond butter, coconut, pumpkin seeds, cinnamon, vanilla, and salt. Stir to combine with large wooden spoon.

6. Transfer mixture to parchment lined pan and firmly press into bottom with hands or spatula. Place in refrigerator for 20 minutes.
7. Remove from refrigerator and cut into bars.
8. Serve chilled. Or allow to warm to room temperature and serve.

Superfood Granola Bowl

Prep Time: 5 minutes

Servings: 1

INGREDIENTS

1/2 cup raw almonds

1/3 cups raw walnuts

1/3 cups cashews

1/4 cup raw pumpkin seeds

1/4 cup shredded or flaked coconut

2 - 3 dried pitted dates

2 tablespoons pomegranate seeds (or goji or noni berries)

1/2 teaspoon Celtic sea salt

Pinch vanilla

Water

INSTRUCTIONS

1. Chop almonds, walnuts and dates by hand. Or add to clean food processor or high-speed blender and pulse to roughly chop.
2. Add to small bowl with pumpkin seeds, coconut, seeds or berries, and vanilla. Mix to combine.
3. Transfer to serving dish and serve immediately. Or store in airtight container.

Skinny Raisin Rugalach

Prep Time: 25 minutes

Cook Time: 20 minutes

Servings: 12

INSTRUCTIONS

Crust

2 cups almond flour

2 cage-free eggs

2 tablespoons coconut oil

2 tablespoons cacao butter (or or coconut butter or coconut cream)

2 tablespoons date butter (or raw honey or agave)

1 teaspoon baking powder

1/2 teaspoon baking soda

1/2 teaspoon vanilla

1/4 teaspoon ground cinnamon

1/4 teaspoon Celtic sea salt

Filling

2/3 cup California raisins

2/3 cup golden raisins

1/4 organic rum (or water)

2 tablespoons date butter (or raw honey or agave)

1/2 teaspoon vanilla

2 teaspoons ground cinnamon

INSTRUCTIONS

1. For *Crust*, sift almond flour into medium mixing bowl. Add baking soda and powder, vanilla, cinnamon and salt.

2. Whisk eggs and date butter in small mixing bowl, then add to flour mixture and combine. Slowly add coconut oil and butter or cream until malleable dough comes together.

3. Roll in plastic wrap or wrap tightly in parchment and refrigerate for 15 minutes.

4. Preheat oven to 350 degrees F. Line sheet pan with parchment or baking mat. Cover cutting board with parchment. Heat medium pan over medium-high heat.

5. For *Filling*, bring 1/4 cup rum or water to simmer In small pot. Add to small heat safe mixing bowl with raisins, vanilla and 1 teaspoon cinnamon. Mix well to combine and set aside about 5 minutes.

6. Remove dough from refrigerator. Roll dough out on parchment covered cutting board to about 1/8 inch thick rectangle with rolling pin.

7. Spread date butter over dough, then sprinkle on remaining 1 teaspoon cinnamon. Stir raisins in bowl again, then sprinkle over dough. Use sharp knife or pizza cutter to cut dough into 12 rectangles.

8. Roll up dough pieces and arrange on prepared sheet pan. Bake for 15 - 20 minutes, or until dough is golden brown and cooked through.

9. Remove from oven and allow to cool about 5 minutes.

10. Serve immediately. Or allow to cool completely and serve room temperature.

Double Chocolate Chip Scone

Prep Time: 10 minutes

Cook Time: 25 minutes

Servings: 8

INGREDIENTS

2 cups almond flour

1/3 cup arrowroot flour

1 cage-free egg

1/4 cup coconut oil (or cacao or coconut butter, melted)

2 tablespoons raw honey (or agave)

2 tablespoons raw cocoa powder

2 teaspoons baking powder

1/2 teaspoon vanilla

1/2 teaspoon Celtic sea salt

1/2 cup organic chocolate chips (or chocolate bark or cacao nibs)

INSTRUCTIONS

1. Preheat oven to 350 degrees F. Line sheet pan with parchment or coat with coconut oil.
2. Whisk together almond flour, arrowroot flour, cocoa, baking powder, salt and vanilla in large mixing bowl.
3. In small mixing bowl, combine egg, and honey with hand mixer or whisk. Beat briskly while slowly pouring in oil or melted butter.
4. Add egg mixture to flour mixture blend and mix until well combined.

5. Roughly chop chocolate bark, if using. Fold in chocolate or cacao nibs until incorporated. Form dough into ball and place on sheet pan . Pat down to flatten to about 1/2 inch thick circle.

6. Cut into eight wedges with pizza cutter or sharp knife. Arrange at least 1 inch apart on prepared sheet pan.

7. Bake for 20 - 25 minutes , or until edges are browned.

8. Remove from oven and let cool completely.

9. Serve room temperature.

Very Berry Fruit Cereal

Prep time: 10 minutes

Cook time: 15 minutes

INGREDIENTS

¼ cup black raspberry

¼ cup raspberry

¼ cup blueberry

¼ cup strawberry

¼ cup water

1 cup buckwheat

1 pomegranate

INSTRUCTIONS:

1. Combine black raspberry, raspberry, blueberry, strawberry and ¼ cup water in a saucepan. Simmer, covered, and stirring occasionally, for 10 minutes.
2. Cook buckwheat according to package directions.
3. Remove seeds from pomegranate, and set seeds in a dish.
4. Spoon some buckwheat into a bowl. Scoop hot berry mixture over the top. Sprinkle pomegranate seeds over the top and serve.

Spicy Kale with Poached Eggs

Prep time: 10 minutes

Cook time: 12 minutes

INGREDIENTS

1 handful kale

2 cage-free eggs

1 small onion

1 clove garlic

1 tbsp extra virgin olive oil

¼ tsp ground black pepper

1 tsp low-sodium horseradish (optional)

INSTRUCTIONS

1. Chop the onion and mince the garlic. De-stem and wash the kale. Leaving a bit of water on the kale is ideal.

2. In a saucepan, add 1 tbsp extra virgin olive oil over medium heat. Add onion and cook until it begins to lose its opaqueness, about 5 minutes.

3. Add kale to saucepan and cover until kale is soft and green, about 5 minutes. Add garlic and stir, then cook another 2 minutes and remove from heat.

4. Fill a saucepan half full of water. Bring the water to a boil, then reduce heat below a boil and hold it there.

5. One by one, crack the eggs into a small cup or bowl and, with the lip of the cup or bowl close to the water's surface, dump the egg

into the water. If necessary, nudge the eggwhites closer to the yolks to keep them together.

6. Once all the eggs are in the water, remove the pan from heat and cover it. Let sit for 4 minutes until all eggs are cooked, then remove eggs from pan.

7. Place the greens on a plate and the two eggs on top of the greens. Top with horseradish if desired. Serve.

Morning Mellow Melon

Prep Time: 5 minutes*

Servings: 1

INGREDIENTS

1 cup honeydew melon (frozen chunks)

1 cup cantaloupe (chunks)

1 grapefruit (about 2/3 cup juice)

2/3 cup thick coconut milk

2 - 4 tablespoons sweetener**

INSTRUCTIONS

1. *Cut honeydew melon flesh away from rind, then cut into chunks and freeze.

2. Cut cantaloupe flesh away from rind, then cut into chunks. Juice grapefruit.

3. Add frozen honeydew chunks and grapefruit juice to high-speed blender. Pulse to break down frozen honeydew.

4. Add remaining ingredients and process until smooth, about 1 minute.

5. Pour into large glass and serve immediately.

**Stevia, dried dates or raw honey*

Bright & Early Orange Whirl

Prep Time: 5 minutes

Servings: 1

INGREDIENTS

1 1/2 cups orange or tangerine juice (about 6 oranges or 10 tangerines)

1/2 cup coconut cream (or thick coconut milk)

2/3 cup ice

1 cage-free egg (optional)

2 tablespoons sweetener* (optional)

INSTRUCTIONS

1. Juice oranges.
2. Add ice and orange juice to high-speed blender. Pulse to crush ice.
3. Add remaining ingredients and process until smooth, about 1 minute.
4. Pour into large glass and serve immediately.

Stevia, dried dates or raw honey

Hearty Apple Almond Salad

Prep Time: 5 minutes

Servings: 1

INSTRUCTIONS

1 apple

1 small banana

1/4 cup blueberries

1/4 cup raw almonds

2 dried pitted dates

2 tablespoons pomegranate seeds (or dried goji or noni berries)

1/4 teaspoon ground cinnamon

INGREDIENTS

1. Core and dice apple. Peel and dice banana. Add to serving dish and mix to combine. Top with blueberries.
2. Chop almonds and dates. Or add to food processor and pulse to coarsely grind.
3. Top fruit with chopped nuts and dates. Sprinkle with pomegranate seeds and cinnamon and serve immediately.

Sweet Citrus Salad with Coconut Cream

Prep Time: 10 minutes

Servings: 1

INSTRUCTIONS

1 fresh coconut (or 1/2 cup flaked coconut)

1/4 - 1/3 cup dried pitted dates (or raw honey)

1 blood orange

1 tangerine (or navel orange or clementine)

1/2 grapefruit (ruby red, pink or white)

1/2 lime

1 tablespoon sunflower seeds (optional)

Water

INGREDIENTS

1. *Soak flaked coconut in 1 cup water overnight in refrigerator, if using. Soak dates in enough water to cover overnight in refrigerator. Drain.

2. Add soaked coconut and soaking liquid to high-speed blender. Or remove flesh from fresh coconut and add to high-speed blender with 3/4 cup water. Process until thick and fairly smooth, about 1 - 2 minutes.

3. Strain mixture through nut milk bag, cheesecloth or strainer back into blender or to food processor.

4. Reserve pulp and set aside to dry and dehydrate, then use as coconut flour.

5. Add soaked dates or honey to processor and process until smooth. Set aside.

6. Peel all citrus and cut into segments. Add to serving dish. Top with sweet coconut cream. Sprinkle on sunflower seeds (optional).

7. Serve immediately. Or refrigerate 20 minutes and serve chilled.

Superfood Breakfast Brownies

Prep Time: 10 minutes

Servings: 2

INGREDIENTS

1 cup dried pitted dates

1/2 cup cashews

1/2 cup sunflower seeds

1/4 cup hulled hemp seeds (or chia or flax seeds)

1/4 cup shredded or flaked coconut

1/4 cup raw cocoa powder

2 tablespoons coconut oil (or coconut butter or cacao butter)

1 teaspoon vanilla

1/4 teaspoon Celtic sea salt

Pinch ground black pepper.

1/4 cup raw cacao nibs (or dried goji berries, noni berries, pomegranates seeds, or any combination)

INSTRUCTIONS

1. Add hemp, chia or flax seeds sunflower seeds to food processor or high-speed blender. Process until finely ground, about 2 minutes. Add sunflower seeds and process until finely ground, about 1 minute. Add cashews and process until finely ground, about 1 minute.

2. Add dates in batches and continue processing until mixture is well ground and sticks together.

3. Add coconut, cocoa , coconut oil, vanilla, salt and pepper. Process about 30 seconds to incorporate.
4. Transfer to medium mixing bowl and add cacao nibs, dried berries or pomegranate seeds. Mix to combine.
5. Transfer mixture to lined loaf pan and press into bottom with hands or spatula. Slice and serve. Or refrigerate 20 minutes to firm, then slice and serve.

Slim 'n' Trim Vegetarian Dishes

Low-Carb Spicy Kale Quiche

Prep time: 10 minutes

Cook time: 15 minutes

Serves: 4

INGREDIENTS

8 cage-free eggs

2 tbsp extra virgin olive oil

1 7oz bag of Kale greens

1 shallot

¼ tsp chipotle chili pepper powder

2 cloves garlic

½ lemon

2 tbsp coconut oil

¼ tbsp ground black pepper

INSTRUCTIONS

1. Place a steamer basket in the bottom of a large pot and fill with water; if you see water rise above the bottom of the basket, pour some out. Bring the water to a boil.
2. Wash the kale and remove the stems. Mince the garlic and shallot and squeeze the juice from the lemon into a bowl.
3. In a large pan, add the eggs and extra virgin olive oil. Mixing in the chipotle chili pepper powder, scramble the eggs, breaking them up until they form many small pieces, tender yet firm.
4. Place the kale in the pot and steam until tender and bright-green.

5. Remove the kale from the pot and combine with the eggs. Add the garlic, shallot and lemon juice, drizzle the coconut oil over top and add the ground black pepper. Mix and stir thoroughly.

6. Serve immediately or chill 20 minutes and then serve.

Eggplant with Pesto Topping

Prep time: 10 minutes

Cook time: 8 minutes

Serves: 4

INGREDIENTS

1 large, thick eggplant

6-8 tomatoes

4 tbsp olive oil

¼ cup fresh basil

2 cloves garlic

INSTRUCTIONS

1. Preheat the grill. Slice the eggplant lengthwise into ½" thick slices, or ensuring that you have 4 slices. Slice the tomatoes into ¼" thick slices. Combine 4 tbsp olive oil with basil and garlic in a food processor and puree together.

2. Grill the eggplant until browned, turning once, about 3-4 minutes per side.

3. Remove eggplant from the grill and lay the tomato slices out over each piece. Top with the pesto puree and serve.

Spicy Zucchini Eggplant Dine

Prep time: 15 minutes

Cook time: 20 minutes

Serves: 4

INGREDIENTS

3 small zucchini

1 eggplant

2 green peppers

6 tomatoes

1 onion

2 medium carrots

1 four-inch sweet orange pepper

1 cup water

1 tbsp extra virgin olive oil

INSTRUCTIONS

1. Using a julienne peeler, peel zucchini, eggplant and green peppers. Green peppers may be too tough for a julienne peeler, in which case try to simulate the effect of one using a knife. Combine the above in a pan with extra virgin olive oil and saute over medium heat, stirring, for 5 minutes.

2. Meanwhile, cut tomatoes into quarters, carrots into ½" thick slices, dice sweet pepper and dice onion. In a saucepan, combine the above with water and cook over medium heat until carrot is tender,

about 15 minutes. Once finished, blend using an immersion blender, or pour into a blender and puree.

3. Pour the sauce over the zucchini, eggplant and peppers and serve.

Lettuce Nut Salad

Prep time: 10 min

Cook time: 6-8 minutes

Serves: 4

INGREDIENTS

1 7oz bag of Romaine lettuce

1 cup strawberries

1 cup blueberries

1 cup kiwi

½ cup almonds

½ cup walnuts

2 cups coconut milk

1 tbsp arrowroot

1 tsp cinnamon

¼ tsp chipotle chili pepper powder

INSTRUCTIONS

1. Dice the fruits. In a saucepan, combine coconut milk, arrowroot, cinnamon and chipotle chili pepper powder over medium heat. Cook, stirring, for 4 minutes. Add the walnuts and almonds to the sauce and continue cooking until slightly thick.
2. Combine lettuce and fruit in a bowl and drizzle the sauce over the top. Serve immediately or chill 20 minutes and then serve.

Eggplant with Red Sauce

Prep time: 10 minutes

Cook time: 8 minutes

Serves: 2

INGREDIENTS

½ large eggplant cut lengthwise

4 asparagus stalks

2 cloves garlic

1 yellow tomato

2 tsp fresh cilantro

2 tbsp extra virgin olive oil

1 cup organic red sauce

INSTRUCTIONS

1. In a medium saucepan, heat the red sauce on low and keep hot.
2. Slice the eggplant into ½ inch slices, 8 slices total. Heat 1 ½ extra virgin olive oil in a frying pan on medium heat. Cook the eggplant two minutes on one side and another two minutes on the other side. Transfer to a plate.
3. Add ½ tbsp to the pan. Slice the garlic. Rinse the asparagus and cut each asparagus stalk into 3 equal lengths.
4. Add garlic and asparagus to pan and sautee until asparagus is tender.
5. Dice yellow tomato and cilantro and mix together.

6. Place four slices of eggplant on each plate. Spoon red sauce over each slice. Cover with tomato/cilantro mixture and evenly distribute asparagus and garlic cloves.
7. Serve.

Sweet Potatoes Roast

Prep time: 10 minutes

Cook time: 30 minutes

INGREDIENTS

3 sweet potatoes

¼ cup extra virgin olive oil

¼ tsp Celtic sea salt

¼ tsp smoked paprika

INSTRUCTIONS

1. Preheat oven to 500 degrees.
2. Peel the potatoes and cut them into small wedges. In a large bowl, combine potato wedges, extra virgin olive oil, Celtic sea salt and smoked paprika. Mix well until all wedges are coated in all ingredients.
3. Place on a baking sheet and bake for 30 minutes, turning once halfway through, and continue cooking until they are well browned.
4. Remove from oven and let cool. Serve.

Pepper Quiche

Prep time: 5 minutes

Cook time: 3-6 minutes

INGREDIENTS

2 cage-free eggs

1 small onion

1 clove garlic

½ red bell pepper

1 tbsp extra virgin olive oil

¼ tsp smoked paprika

¼ tsp ground black pepper

INSTRUCTIONS

1. Finely chop onion, garlic and red bell pepper.
2. Pour extra virgin olive oil into a pan over medium heat.
3. Crack eggs and pour into a small bowl. Combine with onion, garlic and red bell pepper and whisk until mixed together.
4. Pour contents of bowl into pan and add smoked paprika and ground black pepper. Scramble until desired doneness.
5. Serve.

"Green Bean" Casserole

Prep Time: 5 minutes

Cook Time: 20 minutes

Servings: 12

INGREDIENTS

Casserole

4 cups asparagus

2 cups button mushrooms

1 cup nut milk

1/2 cup cegetable stock

2 tablespoons tapioca flour

1 teaspoon ground white pepper (or ground black pepper)

1 teaspoon garlic powder

1 teaspoon onion powder

Crispy Onions

1/2 cup almond meal

1/2 medium onion (yellow or white)

1 cage-free egg

1 teaspoon paprika

1 teaspoon onion powder

1/4 teaspoon ground black pepper

1 teaspoon Celtic sea salt

Coconut oil (for cooking)

INSTRUCTIONS

1. Preheat oven to 350 degrees F. Bring medium pot of water plus 1/2 teaspoon salt to a boil.

2. For *Casserole*, cut asparagus stalks into quarters. Add to boiling water for about 3 - 4 minutes, until tender but not mushy. Drain and shock in ice bath to stop cooking an preserve color. Set aside.

3. Add tapioca flour and vegetable stock to large pan and heat over medium-high heat. Whisk until smooth, then add nut milk, white pepper, garlic and onion powder.

4. Slice mushrooms and add to pan. Stir and thicken about 8 minutes, until thick and creamy.

5. Add asparagus to pan and stir to coat. Pour into baking or casserole dish and bake about 20 minutes, until heated through. Remove from oven and let cool BOUT 5 minutes.

6. Heat medium pan on medium-high heat and coat with coconut oil.

7. For *Crispy Onions*, whisk egg in medium bowl. In shallow dish, mix almond meal with spices.

8. Peel and slice onion. Toss onions in beaten egg, then in seasoned almond meal to coat. Add to hot oiled pan and fry until crispy and golden brown, about 1 - 2 minutes.

9. Drain *Crispy Onions* on paper towel, then sprinkle over *Casserole*. Serve warm.

Mushroom Masala

Prep Time: 10 minutes

Cook Time: 25 minutes

Servings: 8

INGREDIENTS

1 head cauliflower

1 1/2 cups tomato purée (or tomato sauce)

1 pint (2 cups) mushrooms

1 onion

1 chili pepper

1 /2 green bell pepper

1 large garlic clove

1 inch piece fresh ginger

2 teaspoons coriander leaves (optional)

1 teaspoon garam masala

1/2 teaspoon cayenne pepper

1/2 teaspoon ground coriander

1/2 teaspoon Celtic sea salt

3 tablespoons coconut oil or ghee

INSTRUCTIONS

1. Roughly chop cauliflower, then rice cauliflower in food processor, or mince. Add to medium pot with enough water to cover. Heat pot over medium heat and cook until just tender, about 8 minutes. Drain and transfer to serving dish.

2. Heat medium pan over medium heat. Add oil or butter to hot pan.

3. Peel and finely dice onions. Remove seeds, veins and stem from bell pepper and dice. Slice chili pepper. Peel and mince garlic and onion. Add to hot oiled pan and sauté about 5 minutes.

4. Slice mushrooms and add to pan with tomato, salt and spices. Finely chop coriander leaves and add to pan (optional). Sauté and let simmer about 10 - 12 minutes, stirring occasionally.

5. Transfer to serving dish and serve hot with cauliflower rice.

Easy Matzo Ball Soup

Prep Time: 5 minutes*
Cook Time: 10 minutes
Servings: 6

INGREDIENTS

6 cups vegetable stock
2 cups almond flour
4 cage-free egg yolks
1/4 teaspoon ground white pepper (or ground black pepper)
2 teaspoons Celtic sea salt

INSTRUCTIONS

1. In a medium bowl, beat eggs,1 teaspoon salt and pepper until light and frothy, about 2 minutes. Sift almond flour into bowl and mix until dough comes together.
2. *Cover dough with parchment, if preferred, and refrigerate 2 - 4 hours.
3. Add 1 teaspoon salt to large pot of water and bring to boil. Add vegetable stock to medium pot and heat over medium heat.
4. Remove dough from refrigerator and roll into balls. Carefully place dough balls in boiling water. Reduce heat to low, cover and simmer 20 minutes, until cooked through.
5. Transfer matzo balls to serving dish with slotted spoon. Ladle heated vegetable stock over matzo balls and serve hot.

Butternut Squash Soup

Prep Time: 10 minutes

Cook Time: 1 hour

Servings: 4

INGREDIENTS

1 medium-large butternut squash (about 2 cups diced)

2 cups veggie stock

1/2 cup coconut milk (optional)

1/2 onion (white, yellow or sweet)

1/2 large carrot

1/2 celery stalk

1/2 teaspoon ground coriander (optional)

1 cinnamon stick

Ground black pepper, to taste

Celtic sea salt, to taste

2 tablespoons shelled pumpkin seeds (toasted or raw)

2 tablespoons ghee (or coconut oil)

2 tablespoons coconut oil

INSTRUCTIONS

1. Heat oven to 375 degrees F. Heat medium cast iron pan over medium-high heat. Add butter to hot oiled pan.

2. Peel squash and remove seeds. Dice and add to hot oiled pan with salt and pepper, to taste. Sauté until golden, about 3 - 4 minutes.

Place pan in oven and roast until browned on all sides, about 15 minutes.

3. Heat medium pot over medium-low heat. Add coconut oil to hot pot.

4. Peel and dice onion, celery and carrot. Add to hot oiled pot with cinnamon stick, salt and pepper to taste. Sauté until soft but not browned, about 10 minutes.

5. Remove squash from oven and let cool slightly. Add food processor or high-speed blender and process until puréed.

6. Add vegetable broth and coriander (optional) to pot. Increase heat to medium and bring to boil. Simmer about 5 minutes.

7. Stir in squash purée and simmer about 10 minutes. Discard cinnamon stick.

8. Add mixture to food processor or high-speed blender and purée until smooth. Or blend with immerse or stick blender until smooth.

9. Transfer mixture back to hot pot and stir in coconut milk (optional). Transfer to serving dish.

10. Sprinkle with pumpkin seeds and cracked black pepper. Serve hot.

Mexican Tomato Soup

Prep Time: 10 minutes

Cook Time: 40 minutes

Servings: 4

INGREDIENTS

2 cans (14.5 oz) organic crushed tomatoes

2 cans (11.5) organic tomato juice

5 large tomatoes (or 10 plum tomatoes)

1/2 cup coconut milk

1 red bell pepper (or 1/4 cup roasted red peppers, jarred)

1/4 red onion (or yellow or white onion)

2 garlic cloves

1/2 Serrano chili pepper (or other chili pepper) (optional)

1 tablespoon tapioca flour (or arrowroot powder)

2 tablespoons fresh Mexican oregano (or 1 teaspoon dried oregano)

2 large basil leaves

1 teaspoon fresh cracked black pepper (or ground black pepper)

Celtic sea salt, to taste

1 small bunch cilantro (for garnish)

2 tablespoons ghee (or cacao butter, or coconut oil)

INSTRUCTIONS

1. Juice tomatoes and set aside.

2. Roast red bell pepper over stove burner or until broiler, if using. Turn to char on all sides until skins sears. Rub off blackened skin. Cut in half and remove seeds, stem and veins.

3. Heat medium pot over medium-high heat. Add fat to hot pot.

4. Peel onion and garlic. Dice onion, roasted and red pepper. Mince garlic and Serrano pepper (optional). Add to hot oiled pot and sauté until fragrant, about 2 minutes.

5. Add tapioca and coconut milk. Stir to combine. Let cook about 2 minutes.

6. Chiffon (thinly slice) basil. Add to pot with tomato juice, crushed tomatoes, oregano, pepper and salt, to taste. Stir to combine.

7. Bring to simmer, then reduce heat to low. Simmer and reduce about 30 minutes, or until desired consistency is reached.

8. Transfer to serving dish. Chop cilantro and sprinkle over dish for garnish.

9. Serve hot.

Creamy "Cheesy" Broccoli Soup

Prep Time: 10 minutes

Cook Time: 30 minutes

Servings: 4

INGREDIENTS

1 large head broccoli

2 cups vegetable broth

1 cup nut milk

1/2 cup nutritional yeast

1 medium onion (white or yellow)

2 garlic cloves

1 tablespoon coconut aminos (or liquid aminos or tamari)

1 tablespoon mustard powder

Celtic sea salt, to taste.

1 teaspoon ground white pepper (or 1/2 teaspoon ground black pepper)

2 tablespoons bacon fat (or coconut oil, cacao butterr ghee)

Water

INSTRUCTIONS

1. Heat medium pot over medium heat. Add fat or oil to hot pot.
2. Peel onion and garlic. Chop and add to hot pot. Sauté until fragrant, about 2 minutes.
3. Chop broccoli and add to pot with vegetable broth. Increase heat and bring to boil. Cover and boil about 15 - 20 minutes until broccoli is softened.

4. Pour pot in to food processor or high-speed blender with nutritional yeast, coconut aminos, spices and salt, to taste. Process until smooth, about 1 - 2 minutes. Add enough water to reach desired consistency.

5. Transfer to serving dish and serve immediately.

6. Or add back to pot and heat through over medium heat. Then serve.

Pita Bites

Prep Time: *5 minutes

Cook Time: 20 minutes

Servings: 1

INGREDIENTS

Pita Bites

1 cup tapioca flour/starch

1 teaspoon ground chia seed (or flax meal)

1 egg

2 tablespoons coconut oil

1/4 cup water

1/2 teaspoon baking soda

1/4 teaspoon sea salt

Almond Hummus

1 cup skinless almonds

1/3 cup tahini

1 garlic clove

Juice of 1/2 lemon

Zest of 1/2 lemon

1/4 teaspoon sea salt

1/4 cup water

2 tablespoons pine nuts

INSTRUCTIONS

1. *Soak almonds overnight in enough water to cover. Drain and rinse.

2. Preheat oven to 375 degrees F. Cover sheet pan with parchment paper or baking mat. Heat small pot over low heat.

3. For *Pita Bites*, mix 1/3 cup tapioca flour with chia meal, water and 1 tablespoon coconut oil in pot. Stir until mixture comes together. Remove from heat and cool in freezer.

4. In medium bowl, blend remaining tapioca flour, baking soda and salt. Then add egg and remaining oil. Mix until combined.

5. Add cooled chia mixture to bowl and mix to combine. Then remove and knead to form dough.

6. Form large round disk, then use rolling pin to flatten on lined baking sheet. Cut out circles with biscuit cutter or drinking glass, or cut triangles with pizza cutter. Re-roll excess dough and repeat until all dough is used.

7. Arrange pita pieces on sheet pan and place in oven. Bake about 10 minutes. Carefully turn over with spatula and bake another 5 - 7 minutes, or until crisp.

8. Remove from oven and let cool completely. Place in lidded container or sealable lunch bag and serve room temperature.

9. For *Almond Hummus*, add 1/2 of water to all ingredients in food processor or bullet blender and process. Add just enough water to smooth blend.

10. Scrape hummus into lidded container and serve chilled or room temperature with *Pita Bites*.

Simple Gazpacho + Tortilla Chips

Prep Time: 20 minutes

Cook Time: 10 minutes

Servings: 4

INGREDIENTS

Grain-Free Tortillas

Gazpacho

2 (11.5 oz) cans organic tomato juice (or 3 cups juiced tomatoes)

4 plum tomatoes

2 red bell peppers

1 red onion

1 cucumber

3 garlic cloves

1/4 cup apple cider vinegar

1/4 cup coconut oil (or 2 tablespoons coconut oil and 2 tablespoons flavorful oil [walnut, almond, sesame, etc.])

1 teaspoon cracked black pepper (or ground black pepper)

1/2 tablespoon sea salt

INSTRUCTIONS

1. Seed cucumber and tomatoes. Seed, stem and vein bell peppers. Peel onion and garlic. Dice veggies, mince garlic, and add to medium serving bowl.

2. Add tomato juice, vinegar, oil, salt and pepper, and mix well. Place in refrigerator.

3. Heat medium pan over medium-high heat and coat with coconut oil.

4. For *Tortilla Chips*, prepare *Grain-Free Tortillas*.

5. Add more coconut oil to hot pan and allow to heat up. Cut tortillas into wedges with pizza cutter or sharp knife.

6. Add tortilla wedges back to hot pan in single layer and cook about 30 seconds on each side, until golden and crisp. Drain on paper towel. Repeat with remaining tortilla wedges.

7. Transfer warm *Tortilla Chips* to serving dish. Serve immediately with chilled *Gazpacho*.

Grain-Free Tortillas

Prep Time: 5 minutes

Cook Time: 10 minutes

Servings: 2

INGREDIENTS

2 tablespoons almond flour

2 tablespoons coconut flour

1/2 tablespoon flax meal (or ground chia seed)

2 eggs

1/4 cup water (plus extra)

2 tablespoons coconut oil

1/4 teaspoon baking powder

Coconut oil (for cooking)

INSTRUCTIONS

1. Heat medium frying pan over medium-high heat and coat with coconut oil.

2. Whisk together eggs, coconut oil and 1/4 cup water in medium bowl.

3. In separate mixing bowl, blend coconut flour, almond flour, flax or chia seed, and baking powder.

4. Slowly whisk as you pour flourmixture into wet ingredients. If batter appears too thick to spread fairly thin in pan, add up to 4 tablespoon water 1 tablespoon at a time.

5. Use ladle or dry measure cup to pour 1/2 of batter into hot oiled pan. Tilt pan in circular motion as you pour so batter spreads thinly.

6. Cook batter for about 2 minutes or until slightly golden and firm. Flip tortilla with tongs or spatula and cook another 2 minutes. Remove and place on paper towel or parchment.

7. Cook remaining batter for 2 minutes on each side. Re-oil pan as necessary.

8. Fill warm tortillas with meat or veggies of choice and serve warm.

Veggie Burger

Prep Time: 5 minutes

Cook Time: 20 minutes

Servings: 4

INGREDIENTS

Soft Burger Bun

Veggie Burger

2 eggs

1/2 head cauliflower

2 medium carrots

1 small white onion

1 cup walnuts (1/2 cup ground)

1/4 cup almond flour

2 tablespoons tapioca flour

2 tablespoons ground chia seed (or flax meal)

2 cloves garlic

1 teaspoon paprika

1 teaspoon ground black pepper

1 teaspoon sea salt

Topping

1 avocado

1 heirloom tomato

1 white onion

2 ribs romaine lettuce (or preferred lettuce)

INSTRUCTIONS

1. Preheat oven to 350 degrees F. Line sheet pan with parchment paper, or lightly coat with coconut oil. Or lightly coat 6 mini round cake pans with coconut oil.
2. Prepare *Soft Burger Buns* and place in oven.
3. While bread bakes, line dish with parchment paper.
4. Add walnuts and almond four to food processor or bullet blender. Process until finely ground. Add to medium mixing bowl.
5. Peel small onion and garlic. Add to processor or blender with cauliflower and carrots. Process until finely ground. Add eggs, tapioca and chia. Process until mixture becomes thickened and has batter-like consistency.
6. Add veggie mixture and spices to mixing bowl. Mix all ingredients together with hands or wooden spoon until fully combined and uniform.
7. Form veggie mixture into 4 patties and place on parchment lined dish. Place in freezer for 10 minutes.
8. Heat medium skillet over medium-high heat and add 1 tablespoon coconut oil.
9. Peel onion. Make 4 thick slices, keeping full ring intact. Using spatula, place full rings into hot oiled pan. Sear 1 minute on each side. Set aside on paper towel to drain.
10. Reduce heat to medium and coat pan with coconut oil.
11. Remove veggie patties from freezer and place in hot oiled pan. Cook 5 minutes, then carefully flip with spatula and cook another 5 minutes.

12. Remove *Soft Burger Bun* from oven and let cool about 5 minutes.

13. Cut lettuce ribs in half. Cut tomato into 4 thick slices. Slice avocado in half, pit and slice flesh in peel.

14. Slice bun in half and place lettuce on bottom bun, followed by tomato slice. Add burger patty, then grilled onion ring. Finish with a few slices of avocado and top bun.

15. Serve immediately.

Soft Burger Buns

Prep Time: 5 minutes

Cook Time: 15 minutes

Servings: 6

INGREDIENTS

1/4 cup almond flour

1/4 cup coconut flour

4 eggs

2 tablespoons coconut oil

2 tablespoons unsweetened applesauce

1 teaspoon flax meal (or ground chia seed)

1 teaspoon baking powder

1/2 teaspoon sea salt

INSTRUCTIONS

1. Preheat oven to 350 degrees F. Line sheet pan with parchment paper, or lightly coat with coconut oil. Or lightly coat 6 mini round cake pans with coconut oil.

2. Beat eggs, coconut oil and applesauce in medium mixing bowl with hand mixer or whisk.

3. In large mixing bowl, sift together coconut flour, almond flour, flax or chia meal, baking powder and salt. Pour egg mixture into flour mixture and mix until combined.

4. Scoop thick batter onto prepared shcet pan in six 4 inch rounds. Or pour into six prepared mini cake pans for uniformity. Smooth batter with knife or spatula.

5. Place in oven and bake for 12 - 15 minutes, or until tops are firm to the touch and golden.

6. Remove from oven and let cool at least 5 minutes.

7. Slice in half and serve with your favorite patty or filling.

Skinny Egg Salad Sandwich

Prep Time: 5 minutes

Cook Time: 15 minutes

Servings: 2

INGREDIENTS

Sandwich Bread

Avocado Egg Salad

8 eggs

1 avocado

1/4 cup dill pickle relish

3 tablespoons organic mustard

2 teaspoons paprika

1/2 teaspoon ground black pepper

1/4 teaspoon sea salt

INSTRUCTIONS

1. Preheat oven to 350 degrees F. Lightly coat 6 mini round cake pans or medium loaf pan with coconut oil. Bring medium pot of lightly salted water to a boil.
2. Prepare *Sandwich Bread* and place in oven.
3. While bread bakes, gently add eggs to hot water with tongs and cook about 8 - 10 minutes.
4. Drain eggs in colander and run under cold water to cool.

5. While eggs cool, slice and pit avocado. Scoop flesh into medium mixing bowl. Add relish, mustard, salt and spices.

6. Crack eggs shells and peel. Add boiled eggs to medium mixing bowl.

7. Using a fork, mash ingredients together until smooth mixture with soft chunks forms.

8. Remove *Sandwich Bread* from oven and let cool about 5 minutes.

9. Slice bread and fill with *Avocado Egg Salad*.

10. Serve immediately. Or refrigerate about 20 minutes and serve chilled.

Sandwich Bread

Prep Time: 5 minutes

Cook Time: 15 minutes

Servings: 6

INGREDIENTS

2 cups almond flour

4 eggs

1/2 cup coconut cream (or melted cacao butter)

1/2 cup arrowroot powder (or tapioca flour)

1/3 cup ground chia seed (or flax meal)

1/4 cup coconut oil

2 tablespoons unsweetened applesauce

1 teaspoon apple cider vinegar

1 teaspoon baking soda

1/2 teaspoon sea salt

INSTRUCTIONS

1. Preheat oven to 350 degrees F. Lightly coat 6 mini round cake pans with coconut oil.
2. Beat eggs, coconut oil, coconut cream, applesauce and vinegar in medium mixing bowl with hand mixer or whisk.
3. In large mixing bowl, sift together almond flour, arrowroot, chia meal, baking soda and salt. Pour egg mixture into flour mixture and mix until well combined.

4. Pour batter into prepared mini cake pans and bake for about 15 minutes, or until golden brown and toothpick inserted comes out clean.
5. Remove from oven and let cool at least 5 minutes.
6. Slice in half and serve with your favorite deli meats or sandwich salads.

NOTE: Lightly oil medium loaf pan and bake for about 25 minutes for **Sandwich Bread** loaf.

Kelp Noodle Salad

Prep Time: 5 minutes

Cook Time: 5 minutes

Servings: 2

INGREDIENTS

1 package (12 oz) kelp noodles

1/2 lemon

1 small cucumber

1 small red bell pepper

1 large carrot

Small bunch cilantro

2 large basil leaves

Orange Avocado Dressing

1 avocado

1 large orange

1/2 lemon

5 large basil leaves

1/4 teaspoon ground black pepper

1/4 teaspoon cayenne pepper or red pepper flake (optional)

Large bunch cilantro

INSTRUCTIONS

1. Rinse and drain kelp noodles. Add to medium bowl and soak 5 minutes in warm water and juice of 1/2 lemon. Or bring

medium pot of water with juice of 1/2 lemon to a boil and cook kelp noodles for 5 minutes, if softer texture preferred.

2. Peel, seed and cut cucumber in half width-wise. Cut bell pepper in half, then remove stem, seeds and veins. Use vegetable peeler or grater to make long, thin slices of carrot. Thinly slice cucumber and bell pepper lengthwise.

3. Add veggies and drained kelp noodles to medium mixing bowl.

4. For *Orange Avocado Dressing*, add basil and cilantro leaves to food processor or bullet blender with juice of orange and process to break down leaves. Slice avocado in half and remove pit. Scoop flesh into processor with juice of 1/2 lemon, black pepper and hot pepper (optional). Process until thick and until creamy.

5. Pour *Orange Avocado Dressing* over sliced veggies and kelp noodles. Toss to coat.

6. Serve immediately. Or refrigerate for 20 minutes and serve chilled.

Zucchini Salad with Sundried Tomato Sauce

Prep Time: 20 minutes*

Servings: 2

INGREDIENTS

1 medium zucchini

1 tomato

5 sundried tomatoes

1 garlic clove

2 fresh basil leaves

1 tablespoon raw virgin coconut oil (or 2 tablespoons warm water)

1/4 teaspoon ground white pepper (or black pepper)

1/4 teaspoon sea salt

INSTRUCTIONS

1. Run zucchini through spiralizer, slice into long, thin shreds with knife, or use vegetable peeler to make flat, thin slices. Sprinkle with a pinch of salt and pepper, and gently toss to coat.

2. Add tomato, sundried tomatoes, peeled garlic, basil, coconut oil or warm water, and remaining salt and pepper to food processor or bullet blender. Process until sauce of desired consistency forms.

3. Transfer zucchini pasta to serving bowls. Top with tomato sauce and serve immediately.

4. Or refrigerate for 20 minutes and serve chilled.

Quick Raw Avocado Slaw

Prep Time: 10 minutes*

Cook Time: 20 minutes

Servings: 4

INGREDIENTS

1/2 head cabbage (2 cups shredded)

1 avocado

1 carrot

Zest of 1 lemon

Juice of 1 lemon

1 tablespoon raw honey

2 tablespoons apple cider vinegar

1 teaspoon ground white pepper (or black pepper)

1 teaspoon sea salt

INSTRUCTIONS

1. Cut avocado in half and remove pit. Scoop flesh into large mixing bowl and mash with fork.
2. Remove any tough outer leaves and core from cabbage. Shred cabbage and carrot. Add to bowl with vinegar, honey, salt and pepper. Zest *then* juice lemon, and add.
3. Toss to combine.
4. Serve immediately. Or and place in refrigerator for 20 minutes and serve chilled.

Vegetarian Texas Chili

Prep Time: 10 minutes*

Servings: 2

INGREDIENTS

5 - 6 plum tomatoes

1/2 teaspoon dried cumin

1/4 teaspoon chili powder

1/4 teaspoon onion powder

1/4 teaspoon garlic powder

1 teaspoon fresh oregano leaves (or 1/4 teaspoon dried oregano)

1/2 teaspoon ground black pepper

1/4 teaspoon cayenne pepper or red pepper flakes (optional)

1 teaspoon Celtic sea salt

1 teaspoon chia seed (or flax seed)

1/2 cup raw cashews

Water

INSTRUCTIONS

1. *Soak raw cashews in enough water to cover overnight in refrigerator. Drain and rinse. Set aside.

2. Grind chia or flax in food processor or high-speed blender. Set aside.

3. Juice tomatoes. Or add to food processor or high-speed blender and process. Add enough water to reach desired consistency, if necessary. Then strain.

4. Add tomato juice, ground chia or flax, 1/2 of soaked cashews, salt, pepper and spices to blender. Process until smooth, about 1 - 2 minutes.

5. Stir in remaining soaked cashews.

6. Pour into serving bowls and serve immediately.

Skinny Caesar Salad

Prep Time: 10 minutes

Servings: 1

INGREDIENTS

2 cups chopped romaine lettuce

Almond Parmesan

1/4 cup raw almonds

1 teaspoon raw apple cider vinegar

1 teaspoon nutritional yeast (optional)

1/4 teaspoon garlic powder

1/4 teaspoon onion powder

1/4 teaspoon dried oregano

1/4 teaspoon Celtic sea salt

Caesar Dressing

2 tablespoons raw cashews (or raw sunflower seeds)

2 tablespoons raw sunflower seeds

1 tablespoon raw pine nuts (or raw sesame seeds or raw tahini)

2 tablespoons lemon juice

1 teaspoon sweetener*

1 garlic clove

3/4 teaspoon coconut aminos (or nutritional yeast)

1/2 teaspoon dried dill (optional)

Cracked or ground black pepper, to taste

Water

INSTRUCTIONS

1. Rinse, dry and plate romaine lettuce.
2. For *Almond Parmesan*, add almonds, vinegar, salt, spices and nutritional yeast (optional) to food processor or high-speed blender. Process until almonds are coarsely ground and resemble ground parmesan cheese. Set aside.
3. For *Caesar Dressing*, peel garlic and add to food processor or high-speed blender with sweetener and lemon juice. Process until smooth. Then add remaining ingredients and process until smooth, about 1 - 2 minutes. Add enough water to reach desired consistency.
4. Drizzle *Caesar Dressing* over salad and sprinkle with *Almond Parmesan*. Serve immediately.

* *raw honey or dried dates*

Spiced Walnut Autumn Salad

Prep Time: 10 minutes

Servings: 1

INGREDIENTS

Salad

2 cups red lettuce leaves (or other colorful lettuce variety)

1/2 cup arugula

1/2 ripe pear

Spiced Walnuts

1/4 cup walnuts (halves or pieces)

1 tablespoons raw honey (or 1 dried date plus 1 tablespoon water)

1/4 teaspoon ground cinnamon

1/8 teaspoon ground ginger

1/4 teaspoon fresh ground nutmeg

1/8 teaspoon vanilla

1/4 teaspoon ground cardamom (optional)

Orange Vinaigrette

1 orange

2 tablespoons raw apple cider vinegar

2 teaspoons sweetener*

1 teaspoon raw walnut oil (or coconut, almond, sesame oil, etc.)

1 teaspoon raw tahini or sesame seeds (optional)

1 teaspoon ground mustard seeds (or whole mustard seeds)

1/4 teaspoon cracked or ground black pepper

INSTRUCTIONS

1. For *Salad*, rinse, dry and plate lettuce and arugula. Slice pear in half, and remove seeds. Top greens with sliced pears.

2. For *Spiced Walnuts*, process date and water in food processor or high-speed blender until smooth and add to small mixing bowl, if using. Or combine walnuts, spices and raw honey in small mixing bowl. Sprinkle over *Salad*.

3. For *Orange Vinaigrette*, zest and juice orange. Add to food processor or high-speed blender with vinegar, sweetener, spices and tahini (optional) and process until smooth, about 1 minute.

4. Drizzle *Orange Vinaigrette* over salad and serve immediately.

stevia, raw honey or dried dates

Pecan Apricot Spinach Salad

Prep Time: 10 minutes

Servings: 1

INGREDIENTS

Salad

2 cups spinach leaves

1/2 cup chopped kale leaves

4 - 5 dried apricots

3 tablespoons pecans (halves or pieces)

Honey Mustard Vinaigrette

2 tablespoons raw honey (or 2 dried dates + 2 tablespoons water)

2 tablespoons ground mustard (or mustard seed)

2 tablespoons raw apple cider vinegar

3 tablespoons raw oil (coconut, walnut, almond, sesame, etc.)

3/4 teaspoons Celtic sea salt

INSTRUCTIONS

1. For *Salad*, rinse, dry and plate spinach and kale. Chop dried apricots. Sprinkle apricots and pecans over greens.
2. For *Honey Mustard Vinaigrette*, add honey, mustard, vinegar, oil and salt to food processor or high-speed blender and process until smooth, about 1 minute.
3. Drizzle *Honey Mustard Vinaigrette* over salad and serve immediately.

Southern Style Egg Salad

Prep Time: 5 minutes

Cook Time: 15 minutes

Servings: 4

INGREDIENTS

8 cage-free eggs

1 avocado

1 celery stalk

1/4 sweet onion

1/4 cup sweet pickle relish (or dill pickle relish + 1 tablespoon raw honey, agave or date butter)

1/4 cup organic mustard

2 teaspoons paprika

1/2 teaspoon ground black pepper

1/4 teaspoon Celtic sea salt

INSTRUCTIONS

1. Bring medium pot of lightly salted water to a boil. Leave enough room in pot for eggs.

2. Gently add eggs to hot water with tongs and cook about 10 minutes.

3. Drain eggs into colander in sink. Fill pot with cold water and add eggs back to pot. Let cold water run slowly over eggs in pot to cool.

4. Slice and pit avocado. Scoop flesh into medium mixing bowl. Thinly slice celery. Peel and finely dice onion. Add to mixing bowl with relish, mustard, salt and spices. Mix with large spoon to combine.

5. Crack cooled eggs and peel off shells. Add boiled eggs to medium mixing bowl.

6. Use a fork or knife to chop eggs. Use large spoon to mix and mash ingredients together until smooth mixture with soft chunks forms. Stir to combine.

7. Transfer to serving dish and serve immediately. Or refrigerate about 20 minutes and serve chilled.

Pesto Tomato Caprese

Prep Time: 5 minutes

Servings: 2

INGREDIENTS

1 large yellow tomato

1 large red tomato

Small bunch fresh basil

Celtic sea salt, to taste

Crack or ground black pepper, to taste

Basil Pesto

2 cups basil leaves (packed)

1/4 cup raw pine nuts

1/2 - 1/3 cup raw oil (coconut, walnut, almond, sesame, etc.)

2 garlic cloves

1/2 lemon (or 1 tablespoon raw apple cider vinegar)

1/4 teaspoon Celtic sea salt

INSTRUCTIONS

1. For *Basil Pesto*, peel garlic and add to food processor or high-speed blender with squeeze of 1/2 lemon. Process until finely chopped. Add pine nuts, basil, oil and salt and process until finely ground, about 1 minute.
2. Slice tomatoes and plate in alternating colors. Sprinkle with salt and pepper. Chiffon basil leaves.

3. Spread *Basil Pesto* over tomato slices and top with fresh basil. Serve immediately.

Cashew Crunch Kelp Noodle Salad

Prep Time: 10 minutes*

Servings: 2

INGREDIENTS

1 package (12 oz) kelp noodles

1/2 lemon

1/2 small red bell pepper

Cashew Sauce

1 cup raw cashews

1/2 small red bell pepper

1/2 lemon

1 tablespoon coconut aminos (or raw apple cider vinegar)

2 large basil leaves

1/2 teaspoon smoked paprika

1/2 teaspoon ground black pepper

1/2 teaspoon Celtic sea salt

1/4 teaspoon ground turmeric (optional)

1/4 teaspoon smoked chili powder (optional)

Water

INSTRUCTIONS

1. *Soak 3/4 cup cashews in enough water to cover at least 4 hours, or overnight in refrigerator. Drain and rinse.

2. Drain and rinse kelp noodles. Add to medium bowl with warm water and juice of 1/2 lemon. Set aside 5 minutes.

3. Cut bell pepper in half. Remove stem, seeds and veins and set half of pepper aside. Julienne (thinly slice) remaining bell pepper and add to medium mixing bowl.

4. For *Crunchy Cashew Sauce*, add soaked cashews, bell pepper, juice of 1/2 lemon, coconut aminos, basil, salt and spices to food processor or high-speed blender. Process until smooth, about 2 minutes. Add enough water to reach desired consistency. Set aside.

5. Drain kelp noodles and add to sliced bell pepper. Add *Cashew Sauce* and toss to coat. Transfer noodles to serving dishes.

6. Roughly chop remaining 1/4 cup cashews. Sprinkle noodles and serve immediately. Or refrigerate for 20 minutes and serve chilled.

Dill Stuffed Tomatoes

Prep Time: 15 minutes*

Servings: 2

INGREDIENTS

4 medium tomatoes

1 celery stalk

1 small carrot

1 green onion (scallion)

1/3 cup sunflower seeds

1/2 red bell pepper

1/4 small red onion (or sweet onion)

1/2 teaspoon Celtic sea salt

Dill Dressing

1/2 cup raw cashews

1 tablespoon raw apple cider vinegar (or coconut aminos)

1 teaspoon ground mustard (or mustard seeds)

1/2 lemon

1 small garlic clove

2 sprigs fresh dill

1/2 teaspoon Celtic sea salt

1/4 teaspoon ground white pepper (or pinch ground black pepper)

Water

INSTRUCTIONS

1. *Soak cashews in enough water to cover at least 4 hours, or overnight in refrigerator. Drain and rinse.

2. Cut tops off tomatoes and scoop out seeds. Set aside.

3. Finely dice celery and carrot. Slice green onion. Peel and dice onion. Add to medium mixing bowl. Remove stem, seeds and veins from bell pepper, then dice. Add to bowl with sprinkle of salt. Set aside.

4. For *Dill Dressing*, peel garlic and add to food processor or high-speed blender with soaked cashews, vinegar, mustard, squeeze of lemon, dill, salt and pepper. Process until smooth and creamy, about 1 - 2 minutes. Add enough water to reach desired consistency.

5. Pour *Dill Dressing* over chopped veggies. Toss to coat.

6. Plate hollowed tomatoes and stuff with *Dill Dressing* veggie mixture. Serve immediately.

Squash Blossom Stuffers

Prep Time: 10 minutes*

Servings: 4

INGREDIENTS

16 squash blossoms

1/2 cup walnuts

1 avocado

1 small onion

1/2 sprig fresh dill

1/2 lemon

1/2 teaspoon dried thyme

1/2 teaspoon ground white pepper (or ground black pepper)

1/2 teaspoon Celtic sea salt

1 teaspoon dried tarragon (optional)

Water

INSTRUCTIONS

1. *Gently rinse blossoms and pat dry. Let air dry for 30 minutes.
2.   Cut avocado in half and remove pit. Scoop flesh into food processor or high-speed blender with walnuts, dill, squeeze of lemon, salt, pepper and spices. Process until smooth, about 2 minutes. Add enough water to reach desired consistency.
3. Peel onion and mince. Add to small mixing bowl with avocado mixture. Mix to combine.
4. Spoon mixture into squash blossoms. Serve immediately.

Indian Egg Fried Rice

Prep Time: 10 minutes

Cook Time: 15 minutes

Servings: 2

INGREDIENTS

1/2 head cauliflower

4 cage-free eggs

1 small carrot

1/2 red bell pepper

1/2 yellow bell pepper

1/4 onion (yellow or white)

2 small green onions (scallions)

2 tablespoons pure fish sauce (or coconut aminos or liquid aminos)

1 tablespoon coconut aminos (or coconut vinegar or liquid aminos)

1 teaspoon raw honey (or date butter or agave)

1 teaspoon sesame oil (optional)

1 large garlic clove

1/2 piece fresh ginger

1/2 teaspoon red pepper flake

Celtic sea salt, to taste

Coconut oil (for cooking)

Water

INSTRUCTIONS

1. Cut cauliflower into florets and add to food processor with shredding attachment to rice. Or finely mince cauliflower. Set aside.

2. Heat medium pan or wok over high heat. Lightly coat with coconut oil.

3. Whisk eggs in medium mixing bowl. Set aside.

4. Remove stems, seeds and veins from bell peppers, then julienne (thinly slice). Finely dice carrot. Slice green onions. Peel and mince garlic, ginger and onion.

5. Add red pepper flakes to hot oiled pan. Sauté until just cooked fragrant, about 30 seconds. Add garlic, ginger and onion and sauté about 1 minute.

6. Add cauliflower to hot pan. Sauté about 5 minutes, until cauliflower is golden and a bit softened.

7. Add carrot, peppers and 1/2 green onions. Cook another 2 - 5 minutes, until cauliflower is cooked through. Add a few tablespoons of water and cover with lid to steam, if desired.

8. Push veggies aside and make well (opening) in center of pan. Pour whisked eggs into well in center and carefully scramble until fully cooked, about 2 minutes. Mix eggs into veggies.

9. Remove from heat and transfer to serving dish. Sprinkle remaining green onions over dish and serve hot.

Skinny Munchies

Spicy Chicken Wraps

Prep time: 5 minutes

Cook time: 3 minutes

INGREDIENTS

4 slices of chicken deli meat

1 tbsp olive oil

1 small onion

1 red bell pepper

1 avocado

¼ tsp garlic powder

INSTRUCTIONS

1. Remove the nut from the avocado and mash it into a paste. Chop the pepper and onion into small pieces.
2. Combine the garlic powder, pepper and onion in the bowl with the avocado and mix well.
3. Add the olive oil in a pan over low heat and heat the chicken mildly, turning frequently, for 3 minutes.
4. Remove the chicken from heat and place ¼ of the avocado/pepper/onion mixture onto each piece.
5. Wrap the chicken up into tubes and serve.

Fruit Salad

Prep time: 5 minutes

INGREDIENTS

½ banana

1 apple

¼ cup blueberries

½ cup strawberries

¼ cup slivered almonds

1 tbsp raw unfiltered honey

½ tsp cinnamon

INSTRUCTIONS

1. Slice banana, peel core and chop apple, slice strawberries.
2. Combine the fruit in a bowl with slivered almonds. Drizzle with honey and add cinnamon.
3. Serve.

Tahini with Fruit Topping

Prep time: 4 minutes

INGREDIENTS

1 large celery stalk

¼ cup tahini

2 tsp cinnamon

½ cup blueberries

½ cup strawberries

INSTRUCTIONS

1. In a small bowl, mix the cinnamon into the tahini. Wash the celery stalk and dry the concave inside. Chop the strawberries.
2. Spread the tahini mixture throughout the concave inside.
3. Stick the fruit into the tahini side by side alternating blueberry/strawberry.
4. Serve.

Skinny Frozen Coconut

Prep time: 15 minutes

INGREDIENTS

½ cup organic cashew butter

⅓ cup flaked coconut

2 tbsp organic maple syrup

¼ tsp cinnamon

INSTRUCTIONS

1. In a bowl, combine all the ingredients and mix well.
2. Separate into small balls and roll them together in your hands. Place the balls in the fridge for 20 minutes, or in the freezer to make them feel thicker.
3. Serve.

Black Pepper & Kale Chips

Prep time: 15 minutes

Cook time: 10-15 minutes

INGREDIENTS

1 handful baby kale greens

¼ tsp garlic powder

2 tbsp coconut oil

¼ tsp Celtic sea salt

¼ tsp ground black pepper

INSTRUCTIONS

1. Preheat oven to 350 degrees.
2. In a large bowl, combine 2 tbsp melted coconut oil with kale greens, garlic powder, Celtic sea salt and ground black pepper. Mix well.
3. Line a baking sheet with parchment paper and place kale on it. Bake until the edges of the kale are browned, 10-15 minutes.
4. Remove from oven and cool. Serve.

Nuts & Raisin Bars

Prep time: 25 minutes

INGREDIENTS

1 cup cashews

1 cup raisins

¼ tsp cinnamon

⅓ cup shredded coconut

INSTRUCTIONS

1. In a food processor, combine almonds, raisins and cinnamon, and process into a thick butter.
2. Add the coconut flakes and pulse for 15 seconds.
3. Place the mixture on a piece of wax paper and form it into a square. Place this in the freezer for 20 minutes.
4. Cut the square into appropriately-sized pieces. Serve.

Tart Cherry Energy Bar

Prep Time: 25 minutes

Servings: 6

INGREDIENTS

1 cup dried tart cherries

1/4 cup dried pitted dates

1/3 cup warm water

1 lime

1 cup raw almonds

1/4 teaspoon ground ginger

1/4 teaspoon vanilla

1/8 teaspoon Celtic sea salt

INSTRUCTIONS

1. Zest and juice lime into small mixing bowl. Add warm water and dried cherries. Toss to coat and set aside 10 minutes.
2. Line loaf pan with parchment paper.
3. Add nuts and dates to food processor or high-speed blender. Drain soaked cherries and add to processor with cinnamon, vanilla and salt. Process for about 1 minute, until mixture is coarsely ground and sticks together when pressed.
4. Scrape mixture into prepared loaf pan and press firmly into bottom with hands or spatula.
5. Place in refrigerator and chill for 10 minutes. Remove and cut into 6 bars.

6. Serve immediately. Or store in refrigerator up to 2 weeks.

Simple Almond Apricot Balls

Prep Time: 15 minutes

Servings: 12

INGREDIENTS

1/2 cup dried pitted dates

1/3 cup dried apricots

1/3 cup almonds (toasted or roasted, if preferred)

1/4 cup flaked or shredded coconut

1/2 tablespoon raw honey (or agave)

INSTRUCTIONS

1. Add apricots and dates to food processor or high-speed blender. Process until finely chopped, about 1 - 2 minutes.
2. Add almonds and coconut to processor. Process until well ground, about 2 minutes. Add honey and pulse until mixture sticks together, about 30 seconds.
3. Form mixture into 12 balls.
4. Serve immediately. Or store in airtight container in refrigerator up to 2 weeks.

Simple Spiced Honey Nuts

Prep Time: 5 minutes

Cook Time: 5 minutes

Servings: 8

INGREDIENTS

1 cup almonds

1 cup walnuts

1 cup pecans

1 cup hazelnuts (or macadamia nuts)

1/4 cup raw honey (or agave or date butter)

1 teaspoon Celtic sea salt

1 teaspoon paprika (or smoked paprika or Hungarian paprika)

1/2 teaspoon chili powder

1/2 teaspoon ground cumin

1/2 teaspoon ground black pepper

1/2 teaspoon ground ginger

1/2 teaspoon ground cinnamon

1/4 teaspoon vanilla

1/4 teaspoon ground cardamom (optional)

1/4 teaspoon ground clove (optional)

INSTRUCTIONS

1. Heat large cast iron pan or skillet over medium-high heat.
2. Combine salt and spices in small mixing bowl.

3. Add nuts and honey to large mixing bowl and toss to coat. Sprinkle spice mixture over nuts and stir to coat well.

4. Add coated nuts to hot pan and sauté until caramelized, about 5 minutes. Stir continuously and do not burn.

5. Transfer nuts to sheet pan and spread in single layer to cool at least 5 minutes.

6. Transfer to serving dish and serve warm. Or cool completely and serve room temperature.

Zucchini Fries

Prep Time: 15 minutes

Cook Time: 15 minutes

Servings: 2

INGREDIENTS

1 medium zucchini

1 cage-free egg

1/2 cup almond meal

1 teaspoon flax meal (or ground chia seed)

1/2 teaspoon paprika

1 teaspoon ground black pepper

1 teaspoon Celtic sea salt

Coconut oil (for cooking)

INSTRUCTIONS

1. Cut zucchini in half, then slice into 1/3 inch strips. Sprinkle with 1/2 teaspoon salt and place between paper towels to drain excess water. Set aside 10 minutes.

2. Heat large pan over medium-high heat and coat with coconut oil.

3. In a shallow dish, blend almond meal, flax or chia meal, and remaining spices and salt. Beat egg in small mixing bowl.

4. Gently press paper towel to absorb excess moisture from zucchini.

5. In batches, toss zucchini strips in beaten egg to lightly coat, then dredge in seasoned almond meal.

6. Carefully place coated zucchini strips into hot oil and fry about 2 minutes per side, until golden brown and heated through. Turn with tongs half way through cooking.

7. Remove from pan and drain fried on paper towel. Transfer to serving dish.

8. Serve hot with your favorite sauce.

Skinny Jalapeño Lime Hot Wings

Prep Time: 10 minutes

Cook Time: 15 minutes

Servings: 4

INGREDIENTS

12 medium whole chicken wings (about 16 oz)

2 cage-free eggs

1/3 cup almond meal

1 teaspoon flax meal (or ground chia seed)

1/4 teaspoon cayenne pepper

1/2 teaspoon onion powder

1/2 teaspoon garlic powder

1/2 teaspoon smoked paprika

1/2 teaspoon ground black pepper

1/2 teaspoon Celtic sea salt

Jalapeño Lime Sauce

2 medium tomatillos (or green tomatoes)

2 limes

2 tablespoons raw honey (or agave or date butter)

1/2 small bunch cilantro

1/2 onion (yellow, white or red)

2 garlic cloves

1 jalapeño pepper (or other chili pepper)

1/2 teaspoon ground black pepper

1/2 teaspoon cayenne pepper

1/4 teaspoon Celtic sea salt

2 tablespoons coconut oil (optional)

Coconut oil (for cooking)

INSTRUCTIONS

1. Heat large pan over medium-high heat and coat generously with coconut oil.

2. For *Jalapeño Lime Sauce*, peel garlic and onion and add to food processor or high-speed blender. Juice limes into processor. Remove papery outer leaves from tomatillo. Roughly chop and add to processor with cilantro, jalapeño, salt, spices and oil (optional).

3. Process until smooth, about 1 - 2 minutes. Pour into large mixing bowl and set aside.

4. In a shallow dish, blend almond meal, flax or chia meal, spices and salt. Beat eggs in small mixing bowl.

5. Cut chicken wings at joint to separate into winglet and drummet. Lightly coat chicken in seasoned almond meal. Then dip in egg wash to coat. Return to seasoned almond meal and toss to coat well. Gently shake off excess.

6. Carefully place coated chicken wings into hot oil and fry about 2 minutes on each side, until golden brown and cooked through. Turn with tongs half way through cooking.

7. Drain cooked chicken on paper towel, then add to *Jalapeño Lime Sauce* in large mixing bowl. Toss to coat well.

8. Transfer to serving dish and serve hot.

Pancetta Wrapped Shrimp Snacks

Prep Time: 10 minutes

Cook Time: 15 minutes

Servings: 2

INGREDIENTS

12 jumbo shrimp

4 slices nitrate-free pancetta

12 wooden toothpicks

Ground white pepper, to taste

Celtic sea salt, to taste

INSTRUCTIONS

1. Soak toothpicks in water about 5 minutes.
2. Preheat oven to 350 degrees F. Place oven-safe wire rack in sheet pan.
3. Peel and devein shrimp, leaving tail on. Sprinkle with salt and pepper, to taste.
4. Cut pancetta into thirds. Wrap shrimp in pancetta and secure with toothpick.
5. Place wrapped shrimp on wire rack. Bake for about 15 minutes, or until bacon is crisp and shrimp is just cooked through/ Do not overcook.
6. Remove from oven and transfer to serving dish.
7. Serve hot.

Sundried Tomato Cashew Hummus with Carrots

Prep Time: 5 minutes*

Servings: 4

INGREDIENTS

1 1/2 cup raw cashews

1/4 cup sundried tomatoes

1/4 cup raw tahini (or 1/3 cup raw sesame seeds)

1/2 lemon

1 small garlic clove

1 teaspoon ground white pepper (or 1/2 teaspoon ground black pepper)

1/2 teaspoon Celtic sea salt

2 large carrots

Water

INSTRUCTIONS

1. *Soak cashews in enough water to cover at least 4 hours, or overnight in refrigerator. Drain and rinse.
2. Peel garlic. Juice lemon. Add to food processor or high-speed blender with raw sesame seeds and process until smooth, if using.
3. Or add tahini to processor with soaked cashews, sundried tomatoes, garlic, lemon juice, salt and pepper. Process until smooth, about 1 - 2 minutes. Add water or raw oil to reach desired consistency, if necessary.

4. Transfer mixture to serving dish.

5. Peel carrots if desired. Cut into 4 inch long x 1/2 inch thick sticks. Arrange on serving dish.

6. Serve immediately with hummus. Or place in refrigerator for 20 minutes, then serve chilled.

Chocolate Hazelnut Spread with Apples

Prep Time: 5 minutes*

Servings: 2

INGREDIENTS

1 cup raw hazelnuts

1/4 cup raw cocoa powder

1/4 cup raw honey (or dried pitted dates)

2/3 teaspoon vanilla

1/4 teaspoon Celtic sea salt

2 apples

Raw nut milk (optional)

Water

INSTRUCTIONS

1. *Soak hazelnuts in enough water to cover overnight in refrigerator. Soak dates in enough water to cover overnight in refrigerator, if using. Drain and rinse.

2. Add soaked hazelnuts to food processor or high-speed blender and process until smooth, up to 10 minutes. Scrape down sides as needed.

3. Add honey or soaked dates, cocoa powder, vanilla and salt. Process until smooth, about 1 minute. Add nut milk to reach desired consistency, if necessary.

4. Transfer mixture to serving dish.

5. Remove core, seeds and stems from apples. Slice into wedges and arrange on serving dish. Serve immediately.

Chocolate Chia Pudding

Prep Time: 15 minutes

Servings: 2

INGREDIENTS

1 cup nut milk (or 2 mature coconuts + 1 1/2 cups water)

2 - 4 tablespoons raw honey (or dried pitted dates)

2 - 4 tablespoons whole chia seeds

2 - 3 tablespoons cocoa powder

1/2 teaspoon vanilla

INSTRUCTIONS

1. Remove coconut flesh from shells. Add 1 coconut and water to food processor or high-speed blender. Process until well blended and fairly smooth, about 1- 2 minutes.

2. Strain mixture through nut milk bag, cheesecloth or strainer into container. Add coconut milk back to blender with remaining coconut flesh. Process again until well blended and fairly smooth, about 1 minute.

3. Strain mixture through nut milk bag, cheesecloth or strainer into container. Reserve pulp and set aside to dry and dehydrate, then use as coconut flour.

4. Add nut milk to high-speed blender with dates and process until smooth, if using.

5. Or add nut milk to small mixing bowl with honey or stevia, cocoa powder, vanilla and chia seeds. Whisk to combine. Set aside to thicken, about 1 minute.

6. Pour mixture into serving dishes and serve immediately. Or refrigerate 20 minutes and serve chilled.

Holy Loaded Guacamole

Prep Time: 5 minutes

Servings: 2

INGREDIENTS

2 ripe avocados

1 small plum tomato

1/4 small red onion

Medium bunch fresh cilantro

1/2 lime

1/2 teaspoon smoked paprika

1/2 teaspoon ground black pepper

1/2 teaspoon Celtic sea salt

INSTRUCTIONS

1. Cut avocados in half and remove pits. Scoop flesh into small mixing bowl.
2. Peel onion and dice. Dice tomato. Finely chop cilantro. Add to avocado with salt, spices, and squeeze of lime. Mash with fork until well combined.
3. Transfer mixture to serving dish and serve immediately with raw chips. Or refrigerate for 20 minutes and serve chilled.

Bacon Quesadilla

Prep Time: 10 minutes

Cook Time: 20 minutes

Servings: 2

INGREDIENTS

Filling

8 - 12 strips nitrate-free bacon

Tortillas

2 tablespoons almond flour

1 1/2 tablespoons coconut flour

1/2 tablespoon flax meal (or ground chia seed)

1/4 cup water

2 eggs

2 tablespoons coconut oil

1/4 teaspoon baking powder

Coconut oil (for cooking)

Almond Cheese

1 cup skinless almonds*

1/4 cup water

2 tablespoons coconut oil

1 tablespoon lemon juice

1 tablespoon apple cider vinegar

1 garlic clove

1/2 teaspoon sea salt

1/4 teaspoon ground white pepper (or black pepper)

Avocado Cream

1 avocado

1/4 cup full-fat coconut cream

Small bunch cilantro

Juice of half lime

INSTRUCTIONS

1. *For *Almond Cheese*, soak almonds in 1 1/2 cups water overnight. Drain and rinse.

2. Add all *Almond Cheese* ingredients to food processor or bullet blender and process until smooth. Add a few extra tablespoons of water if necessary to achieve thick but smooth consistency. Set aside.

3. Preheat oven to 425 degrees F. Heat medium skillet over medium-high heat.

4. Chop bacon and sauté in skillet until crisp and cooked through, about 5 minutes. Remove bacon and set aside.

5. Reserve half of bacon grease. Add small amount of coconut oil to pan.

6. For *Tortillas*, whisk together eggs, coconut oil and 1/4 cup water in medium bowl. In a separate bowl, blend coconut flour, almond flour, flax or chia seed, and baking powder.

7. Whisk as you slowly pour dry into wet ingredients. If batter appears too thick to spread fairly thin in pan, add up to 4 tablespoons of water 1 tablespoon at a time.

8. Use ladle or dry measure cup to pour 1/2 of batter into hot oiled pan. Tilt pan in circular motion as you pour so batter spreads thinly.

9. Cook batter for about 2 minutes, or until slightly golden and firm. Flip tortilla with tongs or spatula and cook another 2 minutes. Remove and place on paper towel or parchment.

10. Add reserved bacon grease and small amount of coconut oil to pan. Cook remaining batter for 2 minutes on each side.

11. For *Avocado Cream*, slice avocado in half and pit. Scoop flesh into food processor with coconut cream, lime juice and cilantro. Process until smooth. Transfer to serving dish.

12. To assemble quesadilla, spread *Almond Cheese* over both tortillas. Sprinkle one tortilla with crisp bacon and top with other tortilla.

13. Place quesadilla on sheet pan or baking pan. Bake for 5 minutes.

14. Slice quesadilla with sharp knife or pizza cutter. Serve hot with *Avocado Cream*.

Baked Sweet Plantains

Prep Time: 5 minutes

Cook Time: 20 minutes

Servings: 1

INGREDIENTS

1 ripe yellow plantain

1 tablespoon sweetener*

2 tablespoons water

1 teaspoon coconut oil

1/2 teaspoon ground cinnamon

INSTRUCTIONS

1. Preheat oven to 400 degrees F. Line baking pan with parchment, or lightly coat with coconut oil.
2. Cut plantain into 3/4 inch slices. Remove peel from each slice.
3. Toss plantains in small bowl with sweetener, water, oil and cinnamon.
4. Arrange plantains in single layer on baking pan. Bake 10 minutes, then turn over and bake another 10 minutes, or until plantains are golden brown and tender.
5. Serve warm.

raw honey or agave nectar

Ants On A Log

Prep Time: 5 minutes

Cook Time: 5 minutes

Servings: 2

INGREDIENTS

3 celery stalks

2 tablespoons raisins

Cashew Butter

1 cup cashews

1 teaspoon coconut oil

1/2 teaspoon ground cinnamon

INSTRUCTIONS
1. Add cashews, cinnamon, and coconut oil to food processor or bullet blender. Process until smooth. Let mixture rest between periods of processing to reach desired consistency, if necessary.
2. Cut celery stakes into thirds and fill wells with *Cashew Butter*. Place raisins on cashew butter.
3. Serve room temperature. Or refrigerate 10 minutes and serve chilled.

Chocolate Banana Bites

Prep Time: 10 minutes

Cook Time: 5 minutes

Servings: 1

INGREDIENTS

1 banana

2 - 4 oz organic bittersweet or semisweet chocolate

3 tablespoons chopped nuts (or flaked coconut)

DIRECTIONS

1. Heat chocolate over double boiler until melted, about 5 minutes.
2. Peel banana and cut in 1 inch slices.
3. Dip banana pieces into chocolate, or spread chocolate over tops of banana slices.
4. Sprinkle nuts or coconut over chocolate.
5. Place dipped, topped bananas in freezer for 5 minutes, or until chocolate is set.
6. Serve chilled.

NOTE: For *Frozen Chocolate Banana Bites*, leave dipped, topped banana pieces in freezer for 20 minutes, then serve.

Piña Colada Smoothie

Prep Time: 5 minutes

Cook Time: 5 minutes

Servings: 2

INSTRUCTIONS

1 large banana

1 cup pineapple chunks (fresh, frozen or canned)

2 tablespoons flaked coconut

1 cup coconut milk

1 cup ice (crushed preferably)

DIRECTIONS

1. Add banana, pineapple, coconut, coconut milk and ice to highs-speed blender. Process until smooth.
2. Pour into chilled glasses and serve immediately.

Spicy Chicken Bites

Prep Time: 5 minutes

Cook Time: 10 minutes

Servings: 4

INGREDIENTS

8 oz boneless skinless chicken

1/2 cup almond meal

1 teaspoon flax meal

1 teaspoon paprika

1/2 teaspoon cayenne pepper

1/2 teaspoon red pepper flakes

1/2 teaspoon ground black pepper

1/2 teaspoon sea salt

1 egg

1 jalapeño pepper

2 garlic cloves

2 oz organic spicy brown mustard

Coconut oil (for cooking)

INSTRUCTIONS

1. Heat a medium skillet over medium high heat. Lightly coat pan with coconut oil.

2. Slice chicken into 1x1 inch strips. Arrange slices between 2 sheets of parchment and pound with kitchen mallet or rolling pin to flatten slightly. Place flattened pieces between two paper towels to absorb excess moisture.

3. In a shallow dish, blend almond meal, flax meal, dry spices and salt.

4. Add egg , jalapeño and peeled garlic to food processor or bullet blender. Process until fairly smooth. Pour into shallow dish.

5. Dip chicken pieces into jalapeño egg, then dredge in seasoned almond meal.

6. Carefully place coated chicken pieces into hot oil and fry about 2 minutes, until golden brown and cooked through. Turn with tongs half way through.

7. Drain cooked chicken on paper towel, then transfer to serving dish.

8. Serve hot with spicy mustard.

Jalapeño Bacon Bites

Prep Time: 15 minutes

Cook Time: 20 minutes

Servings: 4

INGREDIENTS

6 medium to large jalapeño peppers

6 strips nitrate-free bacon

12 - 24 wooden toothpicks

Nut Cream Cheese

1/2 cup skinless almonds

1/2 cup cashews

2 tablespoons coconut oil

1 tablespoon lemon juice

1 tablespoon apple cider vinegar

1 garlic clove

1/4 teaspoon ground white pepper (or black pepper)

1/2 teaspoon sea salt

INSTRUCTIONS

1. Soak toothpicks in water for about 5 minutes.
2. Peel garlic, and add all *Nut Cream Cheese* ingredients to food processor or bullet blender. Process until smooth. If necessary, let mixture sit for a few minutes, then continue to process to reach desired consistency.

3. Preheat oven to 375 degrees F. Place oven-safe wire rack over sheet pan.

4. Slice jalapeños in half lengthwise. Remove stems, seeds and veins. Cut bacon strips in half.

5. Fill jalapeño wells with *Nut Cream Cheese*, then wrap in half slice of bacon. Use 1 or 2 toothpicks per jalapeño to secure bacon.

6. Place bacon wrapped pepper on wire rack filling side up and place in oven. Bake for about 15 - 20 minutes, or until bacon is crisp. Remove and let cool about 2 minutes.

7. Serve warm or room temperature.

Green Deviled Eggs 'N Ham

Prep Time: 5 minutes

Cook Time: 10 minutes

Servings: 4

INGREDIENTS

8 eggs

1 avocado

1/2 teaspoon ground black pepper

1/2 teaspoon salt

2 oz natural ham

2 tablespoons fresh dill

INSTRUCTIONS

1. Bring medium pot of lightly salted water to boil. Gently add eggs to hot water with tongs and cook about 8 - 10 minutes.
2. Drain eggs in colander and cool in cold water.
3. Crack shells and peel eggs. Cut eggs in half lengthwise and scoop out yolks into small bowl. Arrange whites on platter with center hollows facing up.
4. Mash avocado, salt and pepper with egg yolks until smooth. Dice ham and dill, separately.
5. Scoop avocado blend into each egg white hollow and sprinkle with ham, then dill.
6. Refrigerate about 20 minutes. Serve chilled.

Cocoa Cream Bun

Prep Time: 10 minutes

Cook Time: 20 minutes

Servings: 4

INGREDIENTS

Bun

1 cup tapioca flour/starch

1/4 - 1/3 cup coconut flour

1 egg

1/2 cup warm water

1/2 cup coconut oil

1 tablespoon sweetener*

1 teaspoon apple cider vinegar

1 tablespoon cocoa powder

1/2 teaspoon cinnamon

1/2 teaspoon baking soda

1/2 teaspoon sea salt

Filling

1 cup cashews (raw or roasted)

2 tablespoons coconut cream

2 tablespoons coconut oil

2 tablespoons cocoa powder

3 tablespoons sweetener*

1/2 teaspoon cinnamon

INSTRUCTIONS

1. Preheat oven to 350 degrees F. Line sheet pan with parchment paper or coat with coconut oil. Heat medium skillet over medium-high heat.

2. For *Filling*, add cashews, coconut oil, coconut cream, cocoa powder, sweetener and cinnamon to food processor or bullet blender and process until smooth. Add 1/2 tablespoon coconut oil at a time if needed to reach desired consistency. Set aside.

3. In medium bowl, sift together tapioca flour, 1/4 cup coconut flour, cocoa powder, cinnamon, baking soda and salt. Stir in warm water and oil.

4. Whisk egg in small mixing bowl. Add sweetener and vinegar. Add egg mixture to flour mixture and mix until well combined. Add 1 tablespoon coconut flour or water at a time if needed to form soft and slightly sticky dough.

5. Divide dough into 4 portions and flatten into round disks. Dust your hand or rolling pin with extra tapioca flour to prevent sticking.

6. Scoop *Filling* into center of dough disks and pinch edges of dough together to create round, sealed ball.

7. Place buns sealed side down on sheet pan and pat down slightly. Bake 20 minutes, or until edges are golden brown and dough is cooked through.

8. Serve immediately. Or store in lidded container.

*stevia, raw honey or agave nectar

Chicken Tenders

Prep Time: 5 minutes

Cook Time: 10 minutes

Servings: 2

INGREDIENTS

8 oz boneless, skinless chicken

1 egg

1/2 cup almond meal

1 teaspoon flax meal

1 teaspoon paprika

1/2 teaspoon thyme

1/2 teaspoon onion powder

1/2 teaspoon ground black pepper

1/2 teaspoon sea salt

Honey Mustard

2 tablespoon raw honey or agave nectar

3 tablespoons organic mustard

INSTRUCTIONS

1. Heat a medium skillet over medium high heat. Lightly coat pan with coconut oil.
2. Slice chicken into 1 inch wide strips. Arrange slices between 2 sheets of parchment and pound with kitchen mallet or rolling pin to

flatten slightly. Place flattened pieces between two paper towels to absorb excess moisture.

3. In a shallow dish, blend almond meal, flax meal, spices and salt.

4. Beat egg in small mixing bowl. Dip chicken into beaten egg, then dredge in seasoned almond meal.

5. Carefully place coated chicken strips into hot oil and fry about 3 - 4minutes, until golden brown and cooked through. Turn with tongs half way through cooking.

6. Drain cooked chicken on paper towel, then transfer to serving dish. Serve warm.

7. Or allow to cool and transfer to lidded container. Serve room temperature or chilled.

8. Mix mustard and sweetener in small serving bowl or lidded container. Serve with chicken.

*stevia, raw honey or agave nectar

Homemade Applesauce

Prep Time: 10 minutes

Cook Time: 20 minutes

Servings: 4

INGREDIENTS

2 sweet apples

2 tart apples

1/4 cup sweetener*

3/4 cup water

1/2 teaspoon ground cinnamon

1/4 teaspoon ground ginger

INSTRUCTIONS

1. Peel, core and chop apples. Add to medium pan with sweetener, water and spices. Stir to combine.

2. Cover pan with lid, and heat pan over medium heat. Cook apples about 20 minutes. Transfer to heat-safe bowl and let cool about 5 minutes.

3. Mash apples with fork or potato masher. Then chill in refrigerator.

4. Transfer chilled applesauce to lidded container. Serve chilled or room temperature.

Strawberry Banana Shake

Prep Time: 5 minutes*

Cook Time: 0 minutes

Servings: 1

INGREDIENTS

1 banana

1 cup strawberries

1/2 - 1 cup water

Meat of 1/2 fresh coconut (or 1/2 cup unsweetened flaked or shredded coconut)

INSTRUCTIONS

1. *Soak flaked coconut in water for at least 4 hours.
2. Add fresh or soaked flaked coconut and water to high-speed blender. Process on high until smooth, about 1 minute.
3. Strain coconut mixture through nut milk bag or a few layers of cheese cloth. Squeeze out all excess liquid. Reserve coconut milk. Dry excess coconut, process until finely ground, and use as coconut flour.
4. Remove leaves from strawberries and chop. Peel banana.
5. Add coconut milk to blender with fruit and process on high until smooth.
6. Pour into serving glass and serve immediately.

7. Or chill in refrigerator for 20 minutes, blend for a few seconds to incorporate separated liquid, then pour into serving glass and serve chilled.

Mango Ginger Apple Salad

Prep Time: 5 minutes

Servings: 2

INGREDIENTS

1 ripe mango

1 granny smith apple

1/4 cup raw cashews

1 inch piece fresh ginger

1/2 teaspoon ground ginger

INSTRUCTIONS

1. Slice mango in half around pit. Peel flesh and dice. Add to small mixing bowl.
2. Core apple and dice. Peel ginger and mince. Add to bowl with ground ginger.
3. Roughly chop cashews and add to bowl.
4. Mix well and serve immediately. Or refrigerate 20 minutes and serve chilled.

Tuna Spread

Prep Time: 5 minutes

Servings: 1

INGREDIENTS

7oz (1 can) chunk light tuna

1 avocado

1/2 small red Onion

1 carrot

1 celery stalk

1/2 Lemon

1/2 cucumber

Ground black pepper, to taste

sea salt, to taste

Paprika, to taste

INSTRUCTIONS

1. Drain tuna. Cut celery stalk in half, and preserve larger end. Peel onion. Slice avocado in half, pit and scoop out flesh into small bowl. Mash well.

2. Finely dice onion, smaller half of celery stalk, and carrot. Add to bowl, with spices to taste.

3. Add tuna to bowl, plus squeeze of lemon. Mix until combined and smooth.

4. Slice reserved half of celery stalk into sticks. Slice cucumber into 1/3 inch round.

5. Serve tuna in bowl with cucumber chips and celery sticks.

Slim Mocha Brownie Bites

Prep Time: 5 minutes

Cook Time: 25 minutes

Servings: 16

INGREDIENTS

4 cage-free eggs

1 cup cocoa powder

1/4 cup coconut oil

1/4 cup full-fat coconut milk

1/4 cup sweetener*

2 teaspoons instant espresso (or instant coffee)

1 teaspoon vanilla

INSTRUCTIONS

1. Preheat oven to 350 degrees F. Lightly oil square baking dish or line with parchment.
2. Add eggs, coconut oil, coconut milk and sweetener to medium mixing bowl and beat with hand mixer or whisk. Sift in cocoa powder, espresso and vanilla. Beat until well combined.
3. Pour batter into prepared baking pan and bake for 20 - 25 minutes, until set.
4. Allow to cool completely.
5. Slice and serve room temperature. Or refrigerate and serve chilled.

raw honey, agave nectar or maple syrup

Sea-riously Good Skinny Recipes

New England Clam Chowder

Prep Time: 10 minutes

Cook Time: 40 minutes

Servings: 4

INGREDIENTS

24 - 36 medium live littleneck clams (or other clam varieties)

2 cans (14 oz) full-fat coconut milk

3 - 4 cups clam juice (or fish stock or chicken stock)

4 slices nitrate-free bacon

4 medium parsnips

1 small onion

1 garlic clove

1 tablespoon tapioca flour (or arrow root powder)

1 1/2 teaspoons ground white black pepper (or black pepper)

1 teaspoon Celtic sea salt

Small bunch fresh parsley (for garnish)

Water

INSTRUCTIONS

1. Have fishmonger shuck clams. Or carefully shuck clams yourself. Reserve clam juice. Chop clams, if desired, and add to reserved clam juice. Set aside in refrigerator.

2. Heat medium pot over medium-high heat. Chop bacon and add to hot pot. Sauté until crisp, about 5 - 7 minutes. Stir occasionally.

3. Peel and roughly chop onion. Peel garlic. Add to food processor and pulse until finely chopped, about 1 minute. Or mince. Chop parsnips.

4. Drain bacon on paper towels. Set aside. Reserve bacon fat in hot pot.

5. Add onion, garlic, tapioca salt and pepper to hot oiled pot. Sauté until fragrant, about 2 minutes.

6. Add parsnips. Stir in coconut milk and 2 - 3 cups clam juice. Reduce heat to low and simmer for 20 minutes.

7. Remove clams in their juice from refrigerator and add to pot. Stir in remaining clam juice, if desired. Bring to simmer, then cook another 5 minutes.

8. Transfer to serving dishes. Chop parsley and sprinkle over dish with chopped bacon.

9. Serve immediately.

Calamari with Ginger Sauce

Prep Time: 15 minutes

Cook Time: 20 minutes

Servings: 4

INGREDIENTS

12 oz (3/4) medium whole squid (calamari)

2 cage-free eggs

1/4 cup almond flour

1/4 cup coconut flour

1/4 cup arrowroot powder

1/4 teaspoon Celtic sea salt

Water

Ginger Sauce

1 yellow onion

2 inch piece fresh ginger

1 lemon

1/2 cup coconut vinegar (or apple cider vinegar)

1/2 cup pure fish sauce (or tamari or coconut aminos)

1/2 cup tamari (or coconut aminos or liquid aminos)

INSTRUCTIONS

1. For *Ginger Sauce*, peel and chop ginger and onion. Add to food processor or high-speed blender and process until coarsely ground,

about 1 minute. Add lemon juice, vinegar, fish sauce and tamari. Process until smooth, about 1 minute.

2. Pour mixture into small pot and heat over medium heat. Bring to simmer. Reduce heat to medium-low and cook until *Ginger Sauce* is reduced and thickened, about 10 - 15 minutes. Stir occasionally. Remove from heat and set aside. Then transfer to serving dish.

3. Have fishmonger clean squid. Or remove innards, clean and rinse squid yourself. Then cut into 1/3 inch rings, keeping tentacles intact.

4. Heat medium pan over medium-high heat. Coat pan with about 1/2 inch coconut oil.

5. Add arrowroot to shallow dish. Blend almond flour, coconut, flour and salt to separate shallow dish. Beat eggs and 1 tablespoon water in small mixing bowl or third shallow dish.

6. Dredge calamari rings and tentacles in arrowroot, shaking off excess. Transfer to dish for storage between steps.

7. Dip dusted squid into egg mixture, tossing gently to coat. Shake off excess and place back on dish.

8. Dredge dipped squid in flour mixture and carefully place directly into hot oil. Do not return to dish. Fry about 3 - 5 minutes, until golden brown and just cooked through. Tentacles cook slightly faster than rings. Turn half way through cooking with chopsticks or tongs.

9. Drain calamari on paper towel, then transfer to serving dish.

10. Serve hot with *Ginger Sauce*.

Thai Steamed Mussels

Prep Time: 10 minutes

Cook Time: 10

Servings: 2

INGREDIENTS

2.5 lbs fresh mussels

1/2 can (about 6.5 oz) coconut milk

3 tablespoons dry white wine (or tamari or coconut vinegar)

2 teaspoons Thai red curry paste

1/2 tablespoon pure fish sauce

1/2 tablespoon raw honey (or agave)

2 garlic cloves

1 bunch fresh cilantro

2 limes

INSTRUCTIONS

1. Have fishmonger clean mussels. Or scrub mussels and remove the beards with pliers yourself, if necessary.
2. Juice limes into large pot with lid. Peel and mince garlic. Add to pot with coconut milk, wine, curry paste, fish sauce and honey. Heat over high heat and bring to boil. Stir frequently.
3. Simmer for 1 minute, then add mussels. Cover with lid and cook until mussels open, about 5 - 8 minutes. Sir occasionally.
4. Remove from heat. Chop cilantro and toss with mussels.
5. Transfer mussels and liquid to serving dish. Serve hot.

Chinese Mustard Baked Salmon

Prep Time: 5 minutes

Cook Time: 20 minutes

Servings: 2

INGREDIENTS

2 (8 oz) salmon fillets (deboned, skin-on)

2 cups bok choy or Chinese broccoli (roughly chopped)

1/2 teaspoon sesame seeds

Parchment paper

Kitchen twine

Mustard Sauce

1/4 cup pure fish sauce

2 tablespoons Chinese hot mustard (or Dijon or spicy brown mustard)

1 tablespoon raw honey (or agave)

1 tablespoon tamari (or coconut aminos)

1 tablespoon coconut oil

1/2 lime

1 garlic clove

1/2 inch piece fresh ginger

INSTRUCTIONS

1. Preheat oven to 400 degrees F. Place large sheet pan on bottom rack of oven. Prepare large sheet of parchment.

2. For *Mustard Sauce*, peel and mince garlic and ginger. Add to small mixing bowl with fish sauce, mustard, honey, tamari, coconut oil and lime juice. Mix to combine. Set aside.

3. Chop bok choy or Chinese broccoli and place in the middle of parchment sheet.

4. Place salmon fillets skin-side down over veggies. Brush well with *Mustard Sauce*. Transfer remaining mustard sauce to serving dish.

5. Gather edges of parchment up over salmon and tie tightly with kitchen twine to form sealed pouch.

6. Place pouch directly on hot baking sheet in hot oven. Bake for 20 minutes.

7. Remove from oven and carefully open pouch to release steam. Transfer veggies and salmon to serving dish.

8. Serve hot with remaining *Mustard Sauce*.

Skinny Baked Tilapia Filets

Prep time: 10 minutes

Cook time: 15 minutes

Serves: 4

INGREDIENTS

4 filets of tilapia

¼ tsp chipotle chili pepper powder

1 lemon

1 cup coconut milk

1 clove garlic

1 tsp lemon juice

2 tbsp dill

¼ tsp black ground pepper

INSTRUCTIONS

1. Preheat oven to 350 degrees. Chop the garlic and the dill and cut the lemon into slices.
2. Season tilapia with chipotle chili pepper powder and black ground pepper. Bake for 15 minutes or until tilapia flakes with a fork.
3. Combine coconut milk, garlic, lemon juice and dill in a bowl.
4. Remove fish from oven and pour sauce over the top, placing a lemon wedge over each. Serve immediately or chill 20 minutes and then serve.

Fresh Sashimi Bento Bowl

Prep Time: 20 minutes*

Servings: 1

INGREDIENTS

2 fresh sea scallops (sushi grade)

2 oz fresh salmon filet (sushi grade)

2 oz fresh tuna filet (sushi grade)

1/2 small cucumber

1/2 avocado

1 sheet nori (dried seaweed/sushi paper)

1/2 lemon

1 oz pickled ginger (or 2 inch piece fresh ginger + 2 tablespoons raw apple cider vinegar and 1 tablespoons raw honey)

1 teaspoon real wasabi (or 2 tablespoons fresh ground horseradish)

1/2 teaspoon raw sesame seeds

2 tablespoons salmon roe or caviar (optional)

Sashimi Sauce

2 teaspoons raw sesame oil (or coconut, walnut, almond oil, etc.)

2 teaspoons coconut aminos (or tamari)

1 - 2 teaspoons raw honey

1/2 small scallion

1/2 piece ginger root

INSTRUCTIONS

1. *For fresh pickled ginger, peel ginger and use mandolin, vegetable peeler or slicing attachment on food processor to thinly slice. Add to glass container with vinegar and honey and refrigerate 1 - 7 days.

2. Have fish monger clean and filet tuna and salmon, and remove skin.

3. Place salmon, tuna and scallops in freezer for about 15 minutes to firm.

4. For sashimi sauce, peel ginger and mince. Slice scallion. Add to small mixing bowl with oil, coconut aminos and honey. Transfer to small serving bowl and set aside.

5. Use spiralizer, mandolin or vegetable peeler to thinly slice cucumber, and arrange around serving dish. Cut avocado in half and slice pitted half in peel. Scoop flesh onto serving dish beside fish.

6. Place pickled ginger and wasabi or horse around serving dish.

7. Slice lemon and cut nori into thin strips. Place around serving dish. Place salmon roe or caviar around serving dish (optional).

8. Remove fish from freezer and thinly slice. Arrange fish in center of serving dish. Serve immediately.

Fresh Clams with Cocktail Sauce

Prep Time: 5 minutes*

Servings: 1

INGREDIENTS

12 large little neck clams

3/4 lemon

Raw Cocktail Sauce

1 large tomato

Juice of 1/4 lemon

2 tablespoons raw sesame seeds(or 1 tablespoon raw tahini)

1 tablespoon fresh ground horseradish

Pinch Celtic sea salt

Pinch cracked black pepper

INSTRUCTIONS

1. Have fishmonger shuck clams. *Or carefully shuck clams yourself.
2. Arrange clams around serving dish.
3. Add sesame seeds to food processor or high-speed blender and process until smooth, if using.
4. Or seed tomato and add to processor or blender with tahini, lemon juice, horseradish, salt and pepper. Process until smooth and transfer to small serving bowl.
5. Serving clams with *Raw Cocktail Sauce* immediately.

Asian Shrimp Lettuce Wraps

Prep Time: 35 minutes

Servings: 2

INGREDIENTS

4 large lettuce leaves (thin, flexible ribs)

1 cup cabbage (shredded)

1 small carrot

1/2 green onion

1/2 inch piece fresh ginger

1 small garlic clove

1/2 teaspoon raw sesame seeds

1/2 teaspoon coconut aminos (or tamari or raw apple cider vinegar)

1 teaspoon raw oil (sesame, coconut, walnut, almond, etc.)

Shrimp

10 - 12 medium shrimp

3/4 cup lemon juice (about 5 lemons)

1 teaspoon red pepper flakes

1/2 green onion (scallion)

Almond Sauce

2 tablespoons raw oil (sesame, coconut, walnut, almond, etc.)

1/4 cup raw almond butter (or 1/2 cup raw almonds)

1 tablespoon lemon juice (or coconut aminos or tamari)

1 tablespoons sweetener*

1/2 small mild chili pepper

Water

INSTRUCTIONS

1. For *Shrimp*, slice green onion and reserve half in small mixing bowl. Peel, devein and remove tails from shrimp. Add to separate bowl with lemon juice, remaining green onion and red pepper. Mix to combine. Shrimp should be completely covered in lemon juice. Place in refrigerator for 30 minutes, or until shrimp are opaque.

2. Peel ginger and garlic, and finely grate or mince. Add to green onion with coconut aminos and oil. Mix to combine. Set aside.

3. For *Almond Sauce*, add oil, almond butter or almonds, lemon juice, sweetener and chili pepper to food processor or high-speed blender. Process until smooth and creamy, about 1 - 2 minutes. Add enough water to reach desired consistency. Transfer to serving dish.

4. Shred cabbage and carrot and add to ginger mixture. Toss to coat.

5. Rinse, dry and plate lettuce leaves. Drain shrimp and layer onto lettuce. Top with cabbage mixture and sprinkle on sesame seeds. Roll up lettuce wraps and serve with *Almond Sauce*.

*stevia, raw honey or dried dates

Smoked Salmon Avocado Salad

Prep Time: 10 minutes

Servings: 1

INGREDIENTS

Salad

2 cups soft lettuce leaves (looseleaf or butterhead varieties)

1/2 cup watercress or dandelion leaves (optional)

2 oz smoked salmon

1/2 avocado

1 sprig fresh dill

1 tablespoon caviar (optional)

Avocado Cream Dressing

1/2 avocado

1 sprig fresh dill

1 tablespoon lemon juice

1/2 teaspoon ground black pepper

1/2 teaspoon Celtic sea salt

1/2 coconut

Water

INSTRUCTIONS

1. For *Salad*, rinse, dry and plate lettuce and watercress or dandelion leaves (optional). Cut avocado in half and remover pit. Dice or

slice avocado flesh in peel, then scoop onto greens. Lay smoked salmon over greens.

2. For *Avocado Cream Dressing*, remove coconut flesh from peel and add to food processor or high-speed blender with enough water to reach desired consistency. Process until smooth and creamy, about 1 - 2 minutes. Strain mixture through nut milk bag and place back into blender.

3. Scoop remaining avocado flesh into blender. Add lemon juice, 1 sprig dill, salt and pepper and process until well combined and smooth, about 1 minute.

4. Drizzle *Avocado Cream Dressing* over salad. Mince remaining dill and sprinkle over salad. Dollop caviar over salad (optional).

5. Serve immediately.

stevia, raw honey or dried dates

Tuna Tartar with Avocado and Mango

Prep Time: 15 minutes

Servings: 2

INGREDIENTS

8 oz tuna steak (sushi grade)

1 mango

1 avocado

1 lime

1 garlic clove

Small bunch fresh cilantro

2 tablespoons raw oil (sesame, coconut, almond, walnut, etc.)

1 teaspoon coconut aminos (or raw apple cider vinegar)

1/4 teaspoon red pepper flake

1/4 teaspoon Celtic sea salt

1/4 teaspoon ground pepper

2 tablespoons raw macadamia nuts (optional)

INSTRUCTIONS

1. Add oil, coconut aminos and red pepper flake in small bowl. Cut lime in half and add squeeze of lime. Mix to combine and set aside.

2. Cut avocado in half and remove pit. Dice flesh in peel and scoop into small mixing bowl. Finely chop cilantro. Add to medium mixing bowl with squeeze of remaining lime, salt and pepper. Mix to combine, then set aside.

3. Peel garlic and mince. Cut mango in half around pit. Peel and dice. Add to separate mixing bowl with 1 tablespoon oil and pepper mixture. Toss to coat. Set aside.

4. Dice tuna, discarding any tough white gristle. Finely chop macadamia nuts.

5. Transfer tuna to serving dish. Place in ring mold to form, if preferred. Top with mango and avocado mixtures. Sprinkle on chopped nuts. Drizzle on remaining oil and pepper mixture if preferred.

6. Serve immediately. Or refrigerate 20 minutes and serve chilled.

City Clam Chowder

Prep Time: 35 minutes

Servings: 2

INGREDIENTS

2 dozen live littleneck clams

1 - 1 1/2 cups lemon juice (about 8 lemons)

2 cups tomato juice (about 4 large tomatoes)

2 plum tomatoes

1 celery stalk

1 carrot

1 red bell pepper

1 green bell pepper

1/4 teaspoon cayenne pepper

1/2 teaspoon onion powder

1 teaspoon dried oregano

1 teaspoon dried basil

1 teaspoon ground black pepper

1 teaspoon Celtic sea salt

INSTRUCTIONS

1. Have fishmonger shuck clams. Or carefully shuck clams yourself. Reserve clam juice.

2. Juice lemons into medium mixing bowl. Add clams and toss to coat. Clams should be completely covered in lemon juice. Place in refrigerator for 30 minutes, or until clams are opaque.

3. Juice large tomatoes in juicer then add to food processor or high-speed blender. Or add to food processor or high-speed blender and process, then strain and return to processor.

4. Remove stems, seeds and veins from bell peppers. Cut red and green bell pepper in half. Cut carrot and celery stalks in half. Add half of each veggie to tomato juice with salt and spices. Process until smooth, about 2 minutes. Add to medium mixing bowl. Set aside.

5. Dice plum tomatoes, and remaining celery, carrot, and bell pepper. Add to tomato purée with reserved clam juice, salt and spices.

6. Remove clams from refrigerator and drain lemon juice. Gently rinse, if desired. Add to bowl and mix to combine.

7. Transfer to serving dish and serve immediately.

Salmon Tartar Stack

Prep Time: 10 minutes*

Servings: 2

INGREDIENTS

8 oz boneless, skinless salmon fillet (sushi grade)

2 limes

1 avocado

1 shallot

1 tablespoon raw oil (coconut, walnut, almond, sesame, etc.)

1 teaspoon mustard seeds (or ground mustard)

Medium sprig fresh dill

Celtic sea salt, to taste

Ground black pepper, to taste

2 teaspoons caviar (optional)

INSTRUCTIONS

1. Have fishmonger prepare salmon fillets. Or fillet salmon and remove pin bones and skin.

2. Dice salmon and transfer to serving dish. Top with squeeze of 1/2 lime and sprinkle of salt and pepper. Place in mold to form, if preferred.

3. Peel and thinly slice shallot, then add to small mixing bowl. Juice whole lime into food processor or high-speed blender. Add oil, mustard seeds and pinch of salt and pepper. Process to combine, then add to shallots.

4. Or add lime juice, oil, ground mustard, salt and pepper to shallots. Mix to combine and set aside.

5. Cut avocado in half and remove pit. Dice flesh in peel and scoop into separate mixing bowl. Finely chop dill and add to avocado with squeeze of remaining 1/2 lime, salt and pepper. Mix to combine.

6. Add avocado dill mixture to salmon. Then top with shallot mixture and caviar (optional). Serve immediately.

7. *Or refrigerate 2 hours and serve chilled.

Garlic and White Wine Steamed Mussels

Prep Time: 10 minutes

Cook Time: 5 minutes

Servings: 6

INGREDIENTS

24 fresh green lipped mussels

3 large garlic cloves

1/4 cup ghee (or coconut oil)

1/2 cup white wine (or sparkling apple cider)

1/2 teaspoon sea salt

Medium bunch fresh parsley

INSTRUCTIONS

1. Have fishmonger clean mussels, or scrub mussels and remove the beards with pliers, if necessary.
2. Heat large pan over medium heat. Add ghee or coconut oil and salt.
3. Peel and mince garlic. Add to hot oiled pan and sauté garlic for a few seconds, until aromatic.
4. Add mussels and wine. Cover and cook 3 - 4 minutes, just until most of the mussels open.
5. Remove pan from heat and discard mussels that do not open. Finely chop fresh parsley and add to pan. Toss to combine.
6. Use tongs or slotted spoon to transfer cooked mussels to somewhat deep serving bowl. Pour cooking liquid over mussels.

Shrimp Stuffed Squid

Prep Time: 15 minutes

Cook Time: 25 minutes

Servings: 4

INGREDIENTS

Stuffed Squid

12 medium whole squid (calamari)

8 oz medium shrimp

2 cups baby spinach

1/3 cup almond flour

1 egg

1 tablespoon apple cider vinegar

3 garlic cloves

Small bunch fresh oregano

1/4 teaspoon crushed red pepper flakes

3/4 teaspoon sea salt

2 tablespoons coconut oil

8 wooden toothpicks

Sauce

16 oz (2 cans) organic tomato sauce

1 small onion

2 garlic cloves

1/2 cup dry white wine (or 1/3 cup sparkling apple cider + 3 tablespoons apple cider vinegar)

INSTRUCTIONS

1. Have fishmonger clean squid and peel and devein shrimp. Or clean and rinse squid and peel and devein shrimp yourself.

2. Heat medium pan over medium heat. Add coconut oil to pan.

3. Peel garlic and add to food processor or high-speed blender with shrimp and 4 squid. Pulse until coarse paste forms.

4. Add shrimp paste to medium mixing bowl. Roughly chop spinach and oregano leaves and add to bowl with egg, almond flour, vinegar, red pepper and salt. Mix to combine.

5. Stuff remaining squid bodies with stuffing. Secure closed with toothpicks.

6. Use tongs to add stuffed and secured squid to hot oiled pan. Sear for about 1 minute, then flip.

7. Peel and roughly chop onion and garlic. Add to food processor or high-speed blender with white wine. Process until onion and garlic are well broken down.

8. Pour mixture over seared squid. Add tomato sauce and gently stir to blend. Cover and simmer squid in sauce for 15 minutes.

9. Turn over stuffed squid and continue cooking uncovered another 10 minutes.

10. Remove pan from heat. Remove squid from pan and remove toothpicks from squid with tongs or forks.

11. Transfer squid to serving dish and pour sauce over.

12. Serve hot.

Lobster Newburg

Prep Time: 15 minutes

Cook Time: 25 minutes

Servings: 6

INGREDIENTS

2 (1 lb) live lobsters

2 egg yolks

1/2 cup coconut cream (or kefir + 2 tablespoons sweetener*)

1/4 cup ghee (or cacao butter)

2 tablespoons dry sherry (or 1 tablespoon apple cider vinegar + 1 teaspoon
sweetener*)

1/2 teaspoon sea salt

1/4 teaspoon cayenne pepper

1 /4 teaspoon ground nutmeg

Biscuits

1 1/4 cups almond flour

1 egg

2 tablespoons coconut oil

3/4 teaspoon baking soda

1/8 teaspoon ground white pepper

1/4 teaspoon sea salt

INSTRUCTIONS

1. Preheat oven to 350 degrees F. Line sheet pan with parchment paper. Place 4 ceramic ramekins on parchment, and lightly coat bottom with coconut oil.

2. Bring large pot of salted water to boil. Use tongs to carefully place each lobster in boiling water for just 1 minute. Remove from pot. Crack lobster claws and tails and remove meat. Roughly chop, and set aside.

3. For *Biscuits*, separate egg white into medium bowl, and add yolk to small bowl with coconut oil.

4. Beat egg whites to soft peaks with hand mixer or whisk. Mix yolk and oil, almond flour, baking soda, salt and pepper into egg white to form soft, solid dough.

5. Roll dough into eight balls, then flatten into 1/2-inch thick round biscuits with hands. They should fit ramekins snuggly. Place 1 biscuit at bottom of each ramekin. Set remaining biscuits aside on parchment sheet next to ramekins.

6. In small bowl, whisk together egg yolks and coconut cream until well blended.

7. Melt ghee in medium pan over low heat. Stir in egg mixture and sherry. Stir and cook until mixture thickens slightly, about 5 minutes.

8. Add salt, cayenne and nutmeg. Add par cooked lobster meat and cook about 1 minute then remove from heat.

9. Scoop portion of lobster mixture into each ramekin, over biscuit. Top with remaining biscuit.

10. Place sheet pan in oven and bake 15 minutes, until biscuit is golden and firm on top.

11. Remove from oven and let cool slightly.

12. Serve warm.

raw honey or agave nectar

Seafood Paella

Prep Time: 10 minutes

Cook Time: 25 minutes

Servings: 4

INGREDIENTS

1 large head cauliflower

8 oz chorizo (or other smoked sausage)

8 oz large shrimp

12 live little neck clams

12 live mussels

4 bone-in chicken thighs

1 cup chicken stock (or seafood stock)

1 small white onion

2 tablespoons smoked paprika

1 teaspoon saffron

Pinch ground black pepper

Pinch sea salt

2 tablespoons coconut oil

INSTRUCTIONS

1. Heat large pan over medium heat and add coconut oil.
2. Peel and chop onion. Add to hot oiled pan and sauté until translucent, about 2 minutes.
3. Add chicken thighs and brown about 5 minutes. Turn chicken over and cook another 5 minutes.

4. Rinse and clean clams and mussels, and remove any beards with pliers. Peel and devein shrimp. Cut chorizo into 1 inch slices. Set aside.

5. Roughly chop cauliflower and add to food processor with shredding attachment, process to "rice." Or mince cauliflower with knife.

6. Add riced or minced cauliflower to chicken and sauté 2 minutes. Add chorizo, clams, mussels and shrimp. Add paprika and saffron and sauté another 2 minutes.

7. Add chicken or seafood stock and stir to combine. Increase heat to high and bring to simmer. Reduce heat to medium-high and cover. Let simmer about 5 - 7 minutes, until liquid evaporates, shrimp is opaque, and mussels and clams open. Discard any that do not open.

8. Plate and serve hot.

Skinny Tuna Tartar Crêpes

Prep Time: 5 minutes

Cook Time: 15 minutes

Servings: 4

INGREDIENTS

Crêpes

1 cup tapioca flour

1 cup coconut milk (not full-fat)

1 egg

1/4 teaspoon sea salt

Coconut oil (for cooking)

Tuna Tartar

12 oz tuna steak (sushi grade)

1/4 teaspoon ground white pepper (or ground black pepper)

1/4 teaspoon sea salt

4 tablespoons caviar

Avocado Cream

1 ripe avocado

1/4 cup full-fat coconut oil

2 tablespoons coconut oil

1/4 lemon

INSTRUCTIONS

1. Heat large non-stick pan over medium heat. Coat evenly with coconut oil.
2. For *Crêpes*, blend all ingredients thoroughly in medium bowl with whisk or hand mixer on low speed.
3. When pan is hot, use ladle or dry measure cup to pour in 1/3 cup of crêpe batter while tilting pan in all directions to evenly spread batter.
4. Cook crêpe about 2 minutes, then carefully flip and cook another 1 - 2 minutes.
5. When both sides are lightly browned, transfer crêpe to plate and re-oil pan. Wait until oil is hot to repeat, until remaining batter is cooked.
6. For *Tuna Tartar*, dice tuna and discard any tough white gristle. Add to bowl with salt and pepper. Gently toss with soft spatula or large spoon. Set aside.
7. For *Avocado Cream*, cut avocado in half and remove pit. Scoop flesh into food processor or high-speed blender. Add coconut milk, coconut oil and squeeze of lemon juice. Process until smooth. Add coconut milk or lemon juice to thin to drizzling consistency, if necessary.
8. Add two tablespoons *Avocado Cream* to *Tuna Tartar* and gently toss to coat.
9. Fill crêpes with *Tuna Tartar* down center and fold over each side. Plate fold-side down and drizzle on remaining *Avocado Cream*, to taste. Dollop caviar onto **Crêpes**.
10. Serve immediately.

Smoked Salmon Eggs Benedict

Prep Time: 15 minutes

Cook Time: 25 minutes

Servings: 4

INGREDIENTS

4 cage free eggs

6 oz smoked salmon

2 sprigs fresh dill

English Muffins

1/3 cup coconut flour

1/3 cup almond flour

2 eggs

1/4 cup almond milk (or low-fat coconut milk)

2 tablespoons coconut oil

1/2 teaspoon baking soda

1 teaspoon apple cider vinegar

Hollandaise Sauce

1/2 cup ghee or coconut oil (melted)

2 egg yolks

1/2 lemon

1/4 teaspoon sea salt

INSTRUCTIONS

1. Preheat oven to 400 degrees F. Coat 2 mini-round cake pans or 4-inch diameter ceramic ramekins with coconut oil. Bring medium pot to simmer with 1 teaspoon salt and 1 teaspoon apple cider vinegar.

2. For *English Muffins*, mix baking soda and apple cider vinegar In small bowl. Set aside and allow to froth.

3. In medium mixing bowl, beat egg whites with hand mixer or whisk until thick and frothy. Add yolks, almond and coconut flour, nut milk, and coconut oil. Mix gently.

4. Add baking soda and vinegar mixture to bowl and blend well until smooth and free of clumps.

5. Pour batter into pans or ramekins and place on sheet pan. Place in oven and bake 15 -18 minutes, until golden brown and center is firm to the touch.

6. Crack eggs into 4 separate small bowls. Coat or spray metal ladle with coconut oil. Hold ladle over simmering water and pour 1 egg into coated ladle. Slowly tilt edge of ladle into hot water, filling it gently while keeping ladle just submerged in water. Do not let egg float out of ladle or submerge ladle into water entirely. Hold and cook egg about 1 - 2 minutes, until whites are opaque and yolk is warmed but still runny. Place poached egg on paper towel to drain. Repeat with remaining eggs.

7. Remove muffins from oven. Loosen from sides of cake pans or ramekins with knife and turn out onto wire rack to cool.

8. For *Hollandaise Sauce*, add egg yolks, squeeze of lemon, and salt to food processor or high-speed blender. Processor for 30 seconds. While processor or blender is running, drizzle in melted ghee or

coconut oil very slowly. Process until all fat is added and emulsified and sauce thickens a bit, about 2 minutes.

9. Cut slightly cool *English Muffins* in half and transfer to serving dish.

10. Layer *English Muffin* halves with smoked salmon, then top with a poached egg. Pour *Hollandaise Sauce* over poached eggs, to taste. Sprinkle with pinch of salt and cracked black pepper, if preferred. Chop dill and sprinkle over eggs.

11. Serve immediately.

Seared Tuna Salad

Prep Time: 10 minutes

Cook Time: 10 minutes

Servings: 1

INGREDIENTS

1 cup spinach

1 cup arugula

1 avocado

Seared Tuna

6 oz sushi-grade tuna steak

1 tablespoon sesame oil (or coconut oil)

Juice of 1/2 lemon

1 glove garlic

1/2 inch piece fresh ginger

1 teaspoon sesame seeds

Ginger Glaze

1/2 cup pure fish sauce (or coconut aminos)

1/4 cup apple cider vinegar

Juice of 1 1/2 lemons

2 tablespoons sweetener*

1 inch piece fresh ginger

1 green onion

INSTRUCTIONS

1. For *Ginger Glaze*, peel and grate fresh ginger and slice scallion. Add to small pot with fish sauce, vinegar, sweetener and lemon juice. Heat over medium heat and bring to a simmer. Simmer 5 - 7 minutes, until slightly reduced and thickened. Stir occasionally. Once reduced, transfer to serving dish and refrigerate.

2. For *Seared Tuna*, peel and grate or mince ginger and garlic. Add to small dish with lemon juice and sesame oil and mix to combine. Roll tuna steak in marinade to coat and let sit in dish for 10 minutes in refrigerator.

3. Slice avocado in half and pit. Slice flesh in peel. Place halves together to keep avocado from browning while continuing.

4. Heat small skillet over medium-high heat. Add 1 tablespoon coconut oil.

5. Place marinated tuna in hot oiled pan and sear on each side about 1 minute, until outer flesh is just crisped but inside *is not* cooked through. About 5 minutes.

6. Remove tuna and sprinkle with sesame seeds. Cut tuna into slices.

7. Plate spinach and arugula. Fan out avocado slices over salad.

8. Top salad with *Seared Tuna*. Drizzle on chilled *Ginger Glaze* and serve immediately.

stevia, raw honey or agave nectar

Tilapia Ceviche

Prep Time: 25 minutes

Servings: 4

INGREDIENTS

1 lb fresh, wild caught skinless tilapia fillets

Juice of 4 limes

Juice of 1 lemon

1 plum tomato

1/2 cucumber

1/2 small red onion

Medium bunch cilantro leaves

1/2 teaspoon sea salt

1/2 teaspoon ground black pepper

1 avocado

1 jalapeño pepper (optional)

INSTRUCTIONS

1. Dice fish with sharp knife. Freeze for 20 minutes to make cutting easier and cleaner, if preferred.
2. Add fish to medium mixing bowl. Juice all limes and 1/2 lemon over fish. Gently mix to combine. Cover and chill in refrigerator for 15 to 20 minutes, until fish is opaque.
3. Drain off liquid from fish and discard. Set fish aside.
4. Seed and dice tomato. Peel and dice cucumber and onion. Stem, seed and vein jalapeño pepper, then mince. Finely chop cilantro.

5. Add everything to marinated fish with salt and pepper. Juice remaining 1/2 lemon and mix to combine.

6. Slice avocado in half and pit and slice flesh.

7. Serve *Tilapia Ceviche* immediately with sliced avocado. Or refrigerate for 20 minutes and serve chilled.

Oyster Po' Boy

Prep Time: 15 minutes

Cook Time: 20 minutes

Servings: 2

INGREDIENTS

Long Rolls

12 oysters

1/2 cup coconut flour

1 egg

1 avocado

1 tablespoon lemon juice

1 sprig fresh dill

1 rib lettuce

1 small tomato

8 - 12 dill pickle chips

1/2 teaspoon black pepper

1/2 teaspoon salt

Coconut oil (for cooking)

INSTRUCTIONS

1. Preheat oven to 350 degrees F. Line sheet pan with parchment paper, or lightly coat with coconut oil. Or lightly coat 6 mini loaf pans with coconut oil.
2. Prepare *Long Rolls* and place in oven.

3. Heat small pan over medium heat. Coat with coconut oil.

4. Add coconut flour to small bowl. Beat egg with salt and pepper in separate mixing bowl. Dip each oyster in beaten egg, then dredge in coconut flour.

5. Place each oyster in hot oiled pan and cook until crispy and lightly browned, about 2 minutes on each side.

6. Remove oysters from pan and drain on paper towels.

7. Finely mince dill. Slice and pit avocado. Scoop flesh into small bowl and mix with lemon juice and dill until smooth. Shred lettuce and slice tomatoes.

8. Remove *Long Rolls* from oven and let cool about 2 minutes.

9. Slice rolls along side and spread with avocado mixture. Place shredded lettuce on bottom of bun, then add 6 fried oysters. Top with tomato slices and pickles.

10. Serve immediately.

Long Rolls

Prep Time: 5 minutes

Cook Time: 15 minutes

Servings: 6

INGREDIENTS

1/4 cup almond flour

1/4 cup coconut flour

1/4 cup full-fat coconut milk

3 eggs

2 tablespoons unsweetened applesauce

2 tablespoons tapioca flour (or arrowroot powder)

1 teaspoon baking powder

1/2 teaspoon sea salt

INSTRUCTIONS

1. Preheat oven to 350 degrees F. Line sheet pan with parchment paper, or lightly coat with coconut oil. Or lightly coat 6 mini loaf pans with coconut oil.
2. Beat eggs, coconut milk and applesauce in medium mixing bowl with hand mixer or whisk.
3. In large mixing bowl, sift together coconut flour, almond flour, tapioca or arrowroot, baking powder and salt. Pour egg mixture into flour mixture and mix until combined.

4. Scoop thick batter onto prepared sheet pan in six long forms. Or pour into six prepared mini loaf pans for uniformity. Smooth batter with knife or spatula.

5. Place in oven and bake for 12 - 15 minutes, or until golden and tops are firm to the touch.

6. Remove from oven and let cool at least 5 minutes.

7. Slice in half or split through top, and serve with your favorite link or filling.

Tuna Sandwich

Prep Time: 10 minutes

Cook Time: 15 minutes

Servings: 1

INSTRUCTIONS

Sandwich Bread

7 oz (1 can) chunk light tuna

1/2 avocado

1/2 small red onion

1 small carrot

1 small celery stalk

1/2 small cucumber

1/2 lemon

1/2 teaspoon paprika

1/4 teaspoon cracked black pepper (or ground black pepper)

1/4 teaspoon sea salt

DIRECTIONS
1. Preheat oven to 350 degrees F. Lightly coat 6 mini round cake pans or medium loaf pan with coconut oil. Bring medium pot of lightly salted water to a boil.
2. Prepare *Sandwich Bread* and place in oven.

3. While bread bakes, drain tuna and add to small mixing bowl. Cut celery stalk and carrot in half length-wise. Peel onion and cucumber. Finely dice celery, carrot and onion. Add to bowl.

4. Slice avocado in half and scoop flesh of non-pit half into bowl. Preserve pitted half in airtight container with pit intact for freshness.

5. Add salt, pepper paprika and squeeze of 1/2 lemon into bowl. Mash together with fork until combined and smooth. Slice cucumber into 1/4 inch rounds.

6. Refrigerate tuna mixture if preferred.

7. Remove *Sandwich Bread* from oven and let cool about 5 minutes.

8. Slice bread and fill with tuna mixture. Top with cucumber slices.

9. Serve immediately.

Sandwich Bread

Prep Time: 5 minutes

Cook Time: 15 minutes

Servings: 6

INGREDIENTS

2 cups almond flour

4 eggs

1/2 cup coconut cream (or melted cacao butter)

1/2 cup arrowroot powder (or tapioca flour)

1/3 cup ground chia seed (or flax meal)

1/4 cup coconut oil

2 tablespoons unsweetened applesauce

1 teaspoon apple cider vinegar

1 teaspoon baking soda

1/2 teaspoon sea salt

INSTRUCTIONS

1. Preheat oven to 350 degrees F. Lightly coat 6 mini round cake pans with coconut oil.
2. Beat eggs, coconut oil, coconut cream, applesauce and vinegar in medium mixing bowl with hand mixer or whisk.
3. In large mixing bowl, sift together almond flour, arrowroot, chia meal, baking soda and salt. Pour egg mixture into flour mixture and mix until well combined.

4. Pour batter into prepared mini cake pans and bake for about 15 minutes, or until golden brown and toothpick inserted comes out clean.
5. Remove from oven and let cool at least 5 minutes.
6. Slice in half and serve with your favorite deli meats or sandwich salads.

NOTE: Lightly oil medium loaf pan and bake for about 25 minutes for **Sandwich Bread** loaf.

Healthy Shrimp Taco

Prep Time: 15 minutes

Cook Time: 20 minutes

Servings: 4

INGREDIENTS

Grain-Free Tortillas

Filling

12 oz medium shrimp

1/2 small red onion

1 fresh jalapeño or (2 oz pickled jalapeño)

1 garlic clove

1/2 inch piece ginger root

1/4 head cabbage (1 cup shredded)

Large bunch cilantro

1 avocado

1 tomato

2 limes

Coconut oil (for cooking)

INSTRUCTIONS

1. Heat large pan over medium-high heat and lightly coat with coconut oil.

2. Prepare *Grain-Free Tortillas*, with 4 smaller portions.

3. Keep tortillas warm and moist in oven set to WARM under damp paper towel.

4. Use clean paper towel to carefully wipe out pan. Add 1 tablespoon coconut oil to pan.

5. Peel and devein shrimp, and remove tail. Peel and mince garlic and ginger. Peel and thinly slice onion. Slice fresh jalapeños.

6. Add shrimp to pan with garlic, ginger, onion and jalapeños. Sauté about 2 minutes, then squeeze juice of 1 lime and sprinkle pinch of salt and pepper over shrimp.

7. Sauté shrimp until just cooked, about 5 minutes. Remove from heat.

8. Grate radish, shred cabbage, dice tomato. Slice avocado in half, remove pit, and slice flesh in peel. Chop cilantro.

9. Remove tortillas from oven and layer with sautéed shrimp and onions. Top with shredded cabbage, radish, tomato and avocado slices. Finish with large pinch of cilantro and squeeze of lime.

10. Fold tortillas and serve warm.

Grain-Free Tortillas

Prep Time: 5 minutes

Cook Time: 10 minutes

Servings: 2

INGREDIENTS

2 tablespoons almond flour

2 tablespoons coconut flour

1/2 tablespoon flax meal (or ground chia seed)

2 eggs

1/4 cup water (plus extra)

2 tablespoons coconut oil

1/4 teaspoon baking powder

Coconut oil (for cooking)

INSTRUCTIONS

1. Heat medium frying pan over medium-high heat and coat with coconut oil.

2. Whisk together eggs, coconut oil and 1/4 cup water in medium bowl.

3. In separate mixing bowl, blend coconut flour, almond flour, flax or chia seed, and baking powder.

4. Slowly whisk as you pour flour mixture into wet ingredients. If batter appears too thick to spread fairly thin in pan, add up to 4 tablespoon water 1 tablespoon at a time.

5. Use ladle or dry measure cup to pour 1/2 of batter into hot oiled pan. Tilt pan in circular motion as you pour so batter spreads thinly.

6. Cook batter for about 2 minutes or until slightly golden and firm. Flip tortilla with tongs or spatula and cook another 2 minutes. Remove and place on paper towel or parchment.

7. Cook remaining batter for 2 minutes on each side. Re-oil pan as necessary.

8. Fill warm tortillas with meat or veggies of choice and serve warm.

Coconut Shrimp

Prep Time: 10 minutes

Cook Time: 15 minutes

Servings: 4

INGREDIENTS

3 egg whites

1 lb large shrimp

1 cup flaked coconut

1/2 teaspoon garlic powder

1/2 teaspoon ground white pepper (or ground black pepper)

1 teaspoon sea salt

Coconut oil (for cooking)

Mango Salsa

1 ripe mango

1/2 small white onion

1 small jalapeño

Juice of half lime

INSTRUCTIONS

1. Preheat oven to 425 degrees F. Line sheet pan with parchment paper. Or place oven-safe wire rack over sheet pan.

2. Add coconut to shallow dish.

3. Beat egg whites with salt, pepper and garlic powder in a large mixing bowl with hand mixer or whisk until light and fluffy.

4. Peel and devein shrimp. Leave tails on. Add shrimp to egg whites to coat.

5. Let excess egg white drain from shrimp, then add to coconut flakes. Toss to coat. Return shrimp to egg whites, then coconut flakes again. Press shrimp into coconut and coat well.

6. Place the shrimp on prepared sheet pan. Brush lightly with liquid coconut oil.

7. Place in oven and bake for 5 - 7 minutes. Then turn shrimp over, brush with coconut oil, and bake another 5 - 7 minutes, until coconut is golden brown and shrimp are bright pink.

8. For *Mango Salsa*, slice mango around pit. Peel and dice flesh. Peel and dice onion. Mince jalapeño, discarding seeds and stem. Add to small serving dish juice of half a lime. Mix to combine.

9. Remove shrimp from oven and allow to cool for a few minutes.

10. Serve warm with *Mango Salsa*.

Clams Casino

Prep Time: 5 minutes

Cook Time: 25 minutes

Servings: 4

INGREDIENTS

18 medium littleneck clams

1/3 cup dry white wine (or 1/4 cup sparkling apple cider + 2 tablespoons apple cider vinegar)

4 - 6 slices nitrate-free bacon

1 large red bell pepper

4 shallots

2 large garlic cloves

1/3 cup almonds

1/4 teaspoon dried oregano

1/4 teaspoon ground black pepper

1/4 teaspoon sea salt

2 tablespoons coconut oil

INSTRUCTIONS

1. Have fishmonger shuck clams and loosen meat from bottom shell. Reserve bottom shell.
2. Heat large pan over medium-high heat and add coconut oil. Line sheet pan with parchment or aluminum foil.

3. Finely chop bacon and add to hot pan. Sauté until crisp, about 5 minutes. Use slotted spoon to remove cooked bacon from pan and drain on paper towel. Set aside.

4. Preheat oven to 500 degrees F.

5. Remove seeds, stem and veins from bell pepper, then finely chop. Peel and finely chop shallots. Peel and mince garlic. Add to hot bacon drippings with oregano, salt and pepper. Sauté about 5 minutes, until shallots are tender and translucent.

6. Add wine to pan and simmer until just evaporated, about 2 minutes. Remove pan from heat and stir in reserved bacon.

7. Arrange clams in bottom shells on prepared sheet pan. Spoon bacon mixture onto the clams, packing slightly into mound.

8. Finely chop almonds, or add to food processor or high-speed blender and pulse until finely chopped, with some texture remaining. Sprinkle chopped almonds over clams.

9. Place in oven and bake about 10 minutes, until clams are just cooked through and topping is golden brown and aromatic.

10. Remove from oven and transfer to serving dish.

11. Serve immediately.

Crispy Soft Shell Crab With Garlic Lemon Aioli

Prep Time: 10 minutes

Cook Time: 10 minutes

Servings: 2

INGREDIENTS

2 soft shell crabs

1/4 cup almond flour

2 tablespoons tapioca flour

1 teaspoon paprika

1/4 teaspoon dried oregano

1/4 teaspoon dried thyme

1/4 teaspoon onion powder

1/2 teaspoon garlic powder

1/2 teaspoon black pepper

1/2 teaspoon sea salt

Pinch cayenne pepper (optional)

Coconut oil

Garlic Lemon Aioli

1 garlic clove

1 egg yolk

1/2 lemon

1/8 teaspoon sea salt

1/4 - 2/3 cup coconut oil

INSTRUCTIONS

1. Have fishmonger clean soft-shell crabs. Or clean crabs yourself, then rinse.

2. Heat medium pan over medium-high heat. Coat with coconut oil.

3. Combine almond and tapioca flours with spices in shallow dish. Dredge crabs in seasoned flour mixture.pat flour onto crabs and gently shake off excess.

4. Place coated crabs in hot oiled pan belly-side down. Cook about 5 minutes, until golden and crisp, then flip. Add coconut oil if necessary and cook another 5 minutes, until golden and cooked through. Transfer to paper towel and drain.

5. For *Garlic Lemon Aioli*, peel garlic and add to food processor or high-speed blender with egg yolk, juice of 1/2 lemon and sea salt while crabs cook. Process until garlic is finely ground.

6. Slowly drizzle in enough coconut oil to bring mixture together while running processor. Process until mixture emulsifies and thicken slightly. Transfer to serving dish.

7. Transfer cooked crabs to serving dish and serve immediately with aioli.

Almond Crusted Pan Seared Scallops

Prep Time: 15 minutes

Cook Time:10 minutes

Servings: 2

INGREDIENTS

12 large sea scallops (shelled and cleaned)

1/2 cup organic white wine (or sparkling apple cider)

1/3 cup raw almonds

1 tablespoon ground coriander

1/4 teaspoon fresh ground nutmeg

1/4 teaspoon black pepper

1/2 teaspoon sea Salt

1/2 tablespoon coconut oil

INSTRUCTIONS

1. Preheat oven to 375 degrees F.
2. Add scallops, wine and 1/4 teaspoon salt to small mixing bowl. Set aside to marinate for 10 minutes.
3. Place almonds on dry baking sheet and place in oven. Toast 7 - 8 minutes.
4. Heat medium pan over medium-high heat and add coconut oil.
5. Remove almonds from oven and add to food processor with coriander, nutmeg, 1/4 teaspoon salt and black pepper. Pulse to grind coarsely.

6. Add almond coating to shallow dish. Remove scallops from marinade and coat each side in almond mixture.

7. Place coated scallop in hot oiled pan and grill 2 - 3 minutes on each side.

8. Remove scallops and serve immediately with your favorite greens and vinaigrette.

Basque Style Cod Fish Stew

Prep Time: 30 minutes*

Cook Time: 45 minutes

Servings: 4

INGREDIENTS

8 oz (1/2 lb) salted cod fish

1/2 cup tomato sauce

1/4 cup white wine (or 3 tablespoons white grape juice + 1 tablespoon apple cider vinegar)

2 cage-free eggs

2 large parsnips

1 onion (yellow, red or white)

1 large garlic clove

1/4 cup golden raisins

2 oz roasted red bell peppers (jarred)

2 tablespoons green olives (pitted)

1 teaspoon capers

1 bay leaf

1/4 cup coconut oil

Water

INSTRUCTIONS

1. *Soak salted cod in 2 quarts of water for 8 hours. Change water 3 times throughout soaking time. Drain and cut fish into chunks.

2. Bring small pot of salted water to boil. Hard boil eggs about 10 minutes. Drain and set aside in cold water to cool. Crack and peel shells.

3. Peel onion and garlic. Mince garlic. Slice onion, parsnips, and cooled eggs.

4. In order, layer half of parsnips, cod, onion, eggs, capers, garlic, olives, peppers and raisins in medium pot. Add bay leaf, then half of tomato sauce and coconut oil.

5. In order, layer remaining parsnips, cod, onion, eggs, capers, garlic, olives, peppers and raisins. Add 1 cup water and wine on top. Do not stir.

6. Heat pot over medium heat, cover and bring to a boil. Reduce heat to medium-low and simmer until parsnips are tender, about 30 minutes.

7. Transfer to sourcing dishes and serve immediately.

Delicious Lobster Bisque

Prep Time: 25 minutes

Cook Time: 40 minutes

Servings: 4

INGREDIENTS

16 oz (1 lb) lobster meat (claws and tail from 2 - 3 lobsters)

4 cups vegetable broth

1 can (13.5 oz) full-fat coconut milk (or lite coconut milk)

1 can (6 oz) organic tomato paste

2 tablespoons coconut aminos (apple cider vinegar or liquid aminos)

2 leeks

2 carrots

2 celery stalks

4 large garlic cloves

2 bay leaves

1/2 teaspoon dried basil

1/2 teaspoon dried thyme

1 teaspoon dried oregano

1 teaspoon fresh cracked black pepper (or ground black pepper)

Celtic sea salt, to taste

1 small bunch freash parsley (for garnish)

2 tablespoons ghee (or bacon fat, cacao butter, or coconut oil)

INSTRUCTIONS

1. Chop leeks, carrots and celery. Peel garlic and chop. Add to medium pot with vegetable broth, oregano, basil, thyme, pepper and salt to taste. Add tomato paste and stir to combine. Simmer about 25 minutes.

2. Bring large pot salted water to boil. Boil each lobster about 2 minutes. Let cool, then crack shells and remove meat from claws and tail. Roughly chop and set aside.

3. Pour veggies and broth into food processor or high-speed blender. Process until puréed, about 2 minutes.

4. Add puréed mixture back to pot and heat over medium heat. Bring to simmer and add chopped lobster meat. Stir to combine. Simmer until lobster is cooked through and tender, about 10 minutes.

5. Transfer to serving dish and serve hot.

Red Snapper Soup

Prep Time: 30 minutes

Cook Time: 1 hour

Servings: 4

INGREDIENTS

1 (2 1/2 lbs) whole red snapper (gutted, scaled and cleaned)

2 small onions (yellow, white or red)

3 tomatoes

2 large carrots

4 celery stalks (with leaves)

4 large parsnips

1 medium zucchini cut part-way through, lengthwise

1 lemon

Celtic sea salt, to taste

1/4 cup coconut oil

Water

INSTRUCTIONS

1. Have fishmonger gut, scale and clean fish.
2. Peel and thinly slice onions. Roughly chop carrot, celery and parsnips.
3. Add to large pot with 4 cups water and coconut oil. Bring to a boil over medium heat. Cover and simmer for 15 minutes.

4. Roughly chop tomatoes and zucchini and add to pot. Cover and boil simmer for 20 minutes. Add fish to pot and cover. Simmer for about 25 minutes.

5. Remove from heat. Remove fish and 1/4 veggies from pot and set aside. Squeeze juice of lemon over reserved fish and veggies.

6. Pour remaining veggies and liquid into food processor or high-speed blender. Process until puréed, about 2 minutes.

7. Cut fish into portions. Transfer reserved fish and veggies to serving dish.

8. Pour puréed soup over fish and veggies and serve hot.

Simple Sweet & Savory Bread Recipes

Cheesy Jalapeño "Cornbread"

Prep Time: 5 minutes

Cook Time: 25 minutes

Servings: 12

INGREDIENTS

1 1/2 cups almond flour

3 cage-free eggs

1/2 cup coconut oil (or coconut or cacao butter, melted) (or sub 1/4 cup
with unsweetened applesauce)

1/4 cup nutritional yeast

2 fresh jalapeños (or 1/4 cup pickled jalapeño slices)

2 tablespoons organic apple cider vinegar

2 teaspoons baking powder

1/2 teaspoon paprika

1/2 teaspoon ground turmeric or mustard (optional)

1/2 teaspoon ground white pepper (or ground black pepper)

INSTRUCTIONS

1. Preheat oven to 350 degrees F. Lightly coat baking dish or
   cast-iron pan with coconut oil.

2. Beat eggs in medium mixing bowl with hand mixer or whisk
   until thick and slightly frothy. Add oil or butter, nutritional
   yeast and vinegar. Mix well.

3. Mix in almond meal, baking powder, and spices until
   combined.

4. Remove stems from fresh jalapenos. Slice and remove seeds. Stir in fresh or pickled jalapeño slices.
5. Pour batter into prepared baking dish or pan and bake 30 -35 minutes, until edges are golden brown and top is firm.
6. Remove from oven. Slice and serve warm. Or allow to cool to temperature and serve.

Pure Pumpkin Bread

Prep Time: 5 minutes

Cook Time: 40 minutes

Servings: 8

INGREDIENTS

1 cup almond flour

3/4 cup coconut flour

15 oz (1 can) pumpkin puree

2 cage-free eggs

1/2 cup nut milk

1/2 cup unsweetened applesauce

1/4 cup coconut oil (or coconut or cacao butter, melted) (or nut butter)

1/4 cup raw honey (or agave, date butter or stevia)

1/4 cup pumpkin seeds

2 teaspoons baking soda

1 tablespoon ground cinnamon

1 teaspoon ground nutmeg

1 teaspoon Celtic sea salt

1/2 teaspoon ground black pepper (optional)

Coconut oil (for cooking)

INSTRUCTIONS

1. Preheat oven to 350 degrees F. Coat medium loaf pan with coconut oil.

2. Add eggs, oil or butter, applesauce, nut milk and sweetener to food processor or high-speed blender. Process until thick and light, about 1 - 2 minutes.

3. Add pumpkin, salt and spices. Process to incorporate.

4. Add flour and baking soda to small mixing bowl and stir to combine. Add to processor in batches and process until well combined.

5. Pour batter into prepared loaf pan and bake 35 - 40 minutes, until firm but springy in the center.

6. Remove from oven and set aside to cool.

7. Slice and serve warm. Or allow to cool completely and serve room temperature.

Gluten-Free Poppy Seed Pretzel

Prep Time: 15 minutes

Cook Time: 20 minutes

Servings: 4

INGREDIENTS

1 cup coconut flour

1/2 cup tapioca flour

1/2 cup coconut oil (or cacao or coconut butter)

1/2 cup water

1 cage-free egg

2 tablespoons apple cider vinegar

1/2 teaspoon baking soda

1/2 teaspoon baking powder

Topping

1 tablespoon coconut oil (or full-fat coconut milk)

1 - 2 tablespoons poppy seeds

INSTRUCTIONS

1. Preheat oven to 350 degrees F. Heat medium pan over medium-high heat. Line sheet pan with parchment or baking mat.
2. Add oil or butter, water, vinegar and salt to pot. Bring to a boil and remove from heat.

3. Whisk in tapioca flour. Stir until mixture congeals and comes together.

4. Stir in baking soda and baking powder. Continue mixing for a minute. Mixture will foam and expand. Let mixture sit and cool about 5 minutes.

5. Sift in coconut flour. Mix partially, then beat in egg. Blend until combined. Excess coconut flour may sit in bottom of bowl.

6. Turn out dough onto cutting board dusted with any excess coconut flour from mixture. Knead dough for 2 minutes.

7. Cut dough into 4 equal portions. Roll out pieces into ropes and twist to form classic pretzel twist. Pinch together any crumbled dough.

8. Arrange pretzels on lined sheet pan. For *Topping*, brush with coconut oil or milk and sprinkle generously with poppy seeds.

9. Place sheet pan in oven and bake about 25 minutes, until golden cooked through.

10. Serve warm. Or allow to cool and serve room temperature.

Blueberry Scones

Prep Time: 5 minutes

Cook Time: 25 minutes

Servings: 8

INGREDIENTS

2 cups almond flour

1/3 cup arrowroot powder (or tapioca flour)

1 cage-free egg

1/2 cup dried or frozen blueberries

1/4 cup coconut oil

2 tablespoons sweetener*

2 teaspoons baking powder

1/2 teaspoon vanilla

1/2 teaspoon sea salt

1/4 teaspoon ground cinnamon (optional)

INSTRUCTIONS

1. Preheat oven to 350 degrees F. Line sheet pan with parchment or coat with coconut oil.
2. Whisk together almond flour, arrowroot powder, baking powder, salt, vanilla and cinnamon (optional) in medium mixing bowl.
3. In small mixing bowl, beat egg, oil and sweetener with hand mixer or whisk. Add egg mixture to dry ingredients and mix until well combined.

4. Fold in blueberries. Form dough into ball and place on sheet pan . Pat down to flatten to about 1/2 inch thick circle.

5. Cut into eight wedges with pizza cutter or sharp knife. Arrange at least 1 inch apart on sheet pan and bake for 20 - 25 minutes , or until edges are golden brown.

6. Remove from oven and let cool at least 10 minutes.

7. Serve room temperature.

raw honey, agave nectar or grade B maple syrup

Cinnamon Raisin Bread

Prep Time: 5 minutes

Cook Time: 20 minutes

Servings: 12

INGREDIENTS

3/4 cup coconut flour

3/4 cup almond flour

1/4 cup ground chia seed (or flax meal)

2 cage-free eggs

1/2 cup raisins

1/2 cup coconut oil

1/2 cup unsweetened applesauce

1/4 cup sweetener*

2 tablespoons ground cinnamon

1 teaspoon baking powder

1 teaspoon sea salt

1/2 teaspoon ground black pepper (optional)

INSTRUCTIONS

1. Preheat oven to 350 degrees F. Line baking pan with parchment or coat with coconut oil.
2. In large bowl, whisk eggs with hand mixer or whisk until frothy and light. Add coconut oil, sweetener and applesauce. Blend until combined.

3. Sift coconut and almond flour, chia meal, baking powder, salt and spices into wet ingredients. Beat until smooth and well combined. Stir in raisins.

4. Pour batter into prepared baking pan.

5. Bake for 20 - 25 minutes, or until golden brown and firm to the touch.

6. Remove from oven and let cool about 5 minutes.

7. Slice and serve warm. Or allow to cool completely and serve room temperature.

NOTE: Bake in oiled loaf pan for 40 - 45 minutes for **Cinnamon Raison Bread** loaf.

stevia, raw honey or agave nectar

Skinny Classic Bagels

Prep Time: 10 minutes

Cook Time: 25 minutes

Servings: 8

INGREDIENTS

2 cups almond flour

2 tablespoons coconut flour

2 tablespoons ground chia seed (or flax meal)

1 tablespoon tapioca flour (or arrowroot powder)

4 cage-free eggs

1/3 cup apple cider vinegar

2 tablespoons unsweetened applesauce

2 tablespoons sweetener*

1 teaspoon baking soda

1/2 teaspoon sea salt

INSTRUCTIONS

1. Preheat oven to 350 degrees. Lightly coat donut pan with coconut oil.

2. Add almond, coconut and tapioca flours, chia meal, baking soda and salt to food processor or bullet blender, and process for 1 minute.

3. Add eggs, sweetener, applesauce and apple cider vinegar to flour mixture and process until fully blended, about 1 - 2 minutes.

4. Carefully scoop batter into donut pan, avoiding raised middle.
5. Place in oven and bake about 20 - 25 minutes.
6. Remove and let cool about 5 minutes. Then remove from pan.
7. Slice in half and serve immediately. Or let cool completely and serve room temperature.

NOTE: Bake in 8 round mini cake pans lightly coated with coconut oil if you do not have a donut pan.

stevia, raw honey or agave nectar

Candied Banana Bread

Prep Time: 5 minutes

Cook Time: 25 minutes

Servings: 9

INGREDIENTS

3/4 cup almond flour

1/2 cup coconut flour

2 cage-free eggs

2 overripe bananas

1/4 sweetener*

2 tablespoons coconut oil

1 tablespoons baking powder

1 tablespoon cinnamon

1 teaspoon vanilla

1/2 teaspoon sea salt

2 firm bananas

4 dried pitted dates

1/4 cup water

INSTRUCTIONS

1. Preheat oven to 350 degrees F. Coat square baking pan with coconut oil or line with parchment.

2. Add pitted dates and water to food processor or bullet blender and process until dates are broken down.

3. Add processed dates to medium pan. Heat pan over medium-high heat.

4. Peel and chop firm bananas. Add to hot dates and sauté until caramelized, about 3 minutes. Remove from heat and set aside.

5. In medium mixing bowl, sift flour, baking powder, cinnamon, vanilla and salt.

6. Beat eggs, overripe bananas, coconut oil and sweetener in separate bowl with hand mixer or whisk. Add to flour mixture and mix to combine. Fold in candied bananas.

7. Pour batter into prepared baking pan and bake for about 25 minutes, or until browned and toothpick inserted into center comes out clean.

8. Let cool at least 5 minutes.

9. Slice and serve warm. Or allow to cool completely and serve room temperature.

NOTE: Bake in oiled loaf pan for about 40 minutes for **Candied Banana Bread** Loaf.

stevia, raw honey or agave nectar

Onion Crumpets

Prep Time: 5 minutes

Cook Time: 15 minutes

Servings: 4

INGREDIENTS

1/3 cup coconut flour

4 eggs

1/4 cup nut milk

2 tablespoons coconut oil

1 tablespoon unsweetened applesauce

1/2 teaspoon baking soda

1 teaspoon organic apple cider vinegar

1 teaspoon onion powder

1/4 teaspoon sea salt

1 teaspoon dehydrated onion flakes (optional)

INSTRUCTIONS
1. Preheat oven to 400 degrees F. Coat 4 mini-round cake pans or 4-inch diameter ramekins with coconut oil.
2. In small mixing bowl, mix baking soda and apple cider vinegar. Set aside and allow to froth.
3. In medium bowl, beat eggs with hand mixer or whisk until thick and lightened. Add flour, nut milk, applesauce, onion powder and salt. Mix to combine.

4. Add baking soda and vinegar mixture to medium bowl. Blend well until smooth.

5. Pour batter into prepared pans or ramekins and sprinkle on dehydrated onion flakes (optional). Bake for 12 - 15 minutes, until slightly golden and center is firm to the touch.

6. Remove muffins from oven. Loosen from sides of pans or ramekins with knife, then turn out.

7. Serve warm. Or let cool complete and serve room temperature.

Rosemary Basil Scones

Prep Time: 10 minutes

Cook Time: 25 minutes

Servings: 8

INGREDIENTS

2 cups almond flour

1/3 cup arrowroot flour

1 egg

1/4 cup organic coconut oil

1/2 lemon

2 tablespoons sweetener*

2 teaspoons baking powder

2 sprigs fresh rosemary

 5 - 6 large basil leaves (or 1 1/2 teaspoons dried basil)

1/2 teaspoon vanilla

1/2 teaspoon sea salt

1/4 cup hazelnuts (optional)

INSTRUCTIONS

1. Preheat oven to 350 degrees F. Line sheet pan with parchment or coat with coconut oil.

2. Whisk together flours, baking powder, salt and vanilla in large mixing bowl.

3. Zest 1/2 lemon into small mixing bowl. Finely chop rosemary and chiffon fresh basil. Add herbs to bowl with egg and sweetener.

Beat with hand mixer or whisk while slowly pouring in coconut oil.

4. Add egg mixture to flour blend and mix until well combined.

5. Chop and fold in hazelnuts (optional). Form dough into ball and place on sheet pan. Flatten to 1/2 inch thick circle with hands.

6. Cut into eight wedges with pizza cutter or sharp knife. Arrange at least 1 inch apart on sheet pan and bake for 20 - 25 minutes , or until edges are golden brown.

7. Remove and let cool. Serve room temperature.

* orange juice, raw honey, agave nectar or maple syrup

Fennel Breakfast Biscuits

Prep Time: 5 minutes

Cook Time: 15 minutes

Servings: 8

INGREDIENTS

2 1/2 cups fine almond flour (not almond meal)

2 eggs

1/4 cup coconut oil

2 tablespoons fennel seeds

1 teaspoon baking soda

1/2 teaspoon sea salt

1 tablespoon sweetener*

INSTRUCTIONS

1. Preheat oven to 350 degrees F. Line sheet pan with parchment paper.
2. Grind 1 tablespoon fennels seeds in spice grinder or high-speed blender.
3. Combine almond flour, baking soda, salt and ground fennel in medium bowl.
4. Separate egg whites into separate medium bowl, and yolks into small bowl. Beat egg whites to soft peaks with hand mixer or whisk, about 5 minutes.
5. Mix yolks, oil and sweetener into whites. Mix egg mixture into dry ingredients to form soft, solid dough.

6. Roll dough into balls and flatten into 1 inch round biscuits with hands. Place on prepared sheet pan and brush with coconut oil. Sprinkle on whole fennel seeds.

7. Place in oven for 12 - 15 minutes, until golden and firm on top.

8. Remove from oven and serve warm.

NOTE: Oil square baking pan, gently press in dough, use knife or pizza cutter to score in 9 squares, and bake for about 25 minutes for break-away **Fennel BreakfastPan Biscuits**.

Kefir Sourdough Rolls

Prep Time: 10 minutes*

Cook Time: 20 minutes

Servings: 8

INGREDIENTS

Starter

1 1/3 cups drained kefir milk (no kefir grains left)

1/2 cup almond flour

1/4 cup tapioca flour (or arrowroot powder)

1/2 cup warm water

2 tablespoons sweetener*

Rolls

1/2 cup almond flour

1/2 cup coconut flour

1/4 cup coconut oil

1/2 cup warm water

1 tablespoon apple cider vinegar

1 teaspoon baking soda

1 teaspoon sea salt

INSTRUCTIONS

1. *For *Starter*, add 1/2 cup water to small pot and heat over medium heat until warm. Add all *Starter* ingredients to medium mixing

bowl and mix together. Cover tightly with aluminum foil or parchment paper. Store in a warm area for 12 - 18 hours.

2. Preheat oven to 350 degrees F. Line sheet pan with parchment paper or coat with coconut oil. Or coat muffin pan with coconut oil.

3. For *Rolls*, add 1/2 cup water to small pot and heat over medium heat until warm. Sift almond flour, coconut flour, baking soda and salt into Starter. Add coconut oil and vinegar and mix to combine. Add enough warm water to form sticky dough.

4. Shape dough into rolls with hands and place on prepared sheet pan, or scoop into muffin pan.

5. Place in oven for 15 - 20 minute, until golden brown and cooked through.

6. Remove from oven and serve warm. Or allow to cool completely and serve room temperature.

* raw honey or agave nectar

Everything Bagels

Prep Time:10 minutes

Cook Time: 25 minutes

Servings: 8

INGREDIENTS

2 cups almond flour

2 tablespoons coconut flour

4 eggs

1/3 cup apple cider vinegar

2 tablespoons sweetener*

2 tablespoons unsweetened applesauce

2 tablespoons ground chia seed (or flax meal)

1 tablespoon tapioca flour (or arrowroot powder)

1 teaspoon baking soda

1 teaspoon garlic powder

1 teaspoon onion powder

1 teaspoon poppy seeds

1 teaspoon sesame seeds

1 teaspoon caraway seeds (optional)

1/2 teaspoon sea salt

INSTRUCTIONS

1. Preheat oven to 350 degrees F. Lightly coat donut pan with coconut oil.

2. Add flours, chia or flax meal, baking soda and salt to food processor or high-speed blender. Process for 1 minute, until very fine.

3. Add eggs, sweetener, applesauce, vinegar, salt and spices to flour mixture. Process until fully blended, about 1 - 2 minutes.

4. Carefully scoop batter into donut pan, avoiding raised middle. Sprinkle on poppy, sesame and caraway seeds (optional).

5. Place in oven and bake for 20 - 25 minutes.

6. Remove at let cool about 5 minutes. Then remove bagels from pan.

7. Serve immediately Or let cool completely and serve room temperature.

NOTE: Bake in 8 round mini cake pans lightly coated with coconut oil if you do not have a donut pan.

* stevia, raw honey or agave nectar

Skinny Egg Bread

Prep Time: 15 minutes

Cook Time: 20 minutes

Servings: 4

INGREDIENTS

3 cups almond flour

6 egg yolks (room temperature)

3 eggs (room temperature)

1/2 cup coconut oil

1/4 cup sweetener*

1 tablespoon apple cider vinegar

1 teaspoon baking soda

1/2 teaspoon sea salt

1 egg

INSTRUCTIONS

1. Preheat oven to 350 degrees F. Coat muffin pan with coconut oil or line with paper liners. Cover cutting board with parchment.

2. Add eggs and yolks to large mixing bowl. Beat with hand mixer or whisk until light and frothy. Beat in coconut oil, sweetener, vinegar, baking soda and salt. Sift in 2 1/2 cups almond flower while mixing to form sticky dough.

3. Dust parchment covered cutting board with remaining almond flour. Turn dough out onto parchment and knead for about 5 minutes.

4. Transfer dough to prepared muffin pan. Beat remaining egg in small mixing bowl and brush over bread.

5. Place in oven and bake 15 - 20 minutes, until browned and cooked through.

6. Remove from oven and let cool for 5 minutes.

7. Serve warm. Or allow to cool completely and serve room temperature.

Cocoa Gingerbread

Prep Time: 5 minutes

Cook Time: 20 minutes

Servings: 8

INGREDIENTS

2 cups almond flour

2 tablespoons ground chia seed (or flax meal)

2 eggs

1/2 cup unsweetened applesauce

1/4 cup coconut oil

1/4 cup sweetener*

1/4 cup cocoa powder

1 tablespoon baking powder

1 teaspoon baking soda

2 tablespoons ground ginger

1 tablespoon ground cinnamon

1 teaspoon ground black pepper

1 teaspoon vanilla

1/2 teaspoon ground cloves

2 oz fresh ginger juice (optional)

INSTRUCTIONS

1. Preheat oven to 350 degrees F. Coat 2 small loaf pans with coconut oil.

2. Beat eggs in large mixing bowl with hand mixer or whisk until light and thickened, about 2 minutes. Add applesauce, oil, sweetener and ginger juice (optional). Beat well.

3. Sift all dry ingredients Into medium mixing bowl. Slowly beat flour mixture into egg mixture.

4. Pour batter into prepared loaf pans and bake for 20 - 25 minutes, or until toothpick inserted into center comes out clean.

5. Let cool at least 5 minutes. Insert knife around edges and remove brad from pan.

6. Slice and serve warm. Or let cool completely and serve room temperature.

NOTE: Bake in large oiled loaf pan for 35 - 45 minutes for **Cocoa Gingerbread Loaf**.

raw honey, agave nectar, maple syrup, molasses

Apple Bread

Prep Time: 10 minutes

Cook Time: 20 minutes

Servings: 24

INGREDIENTS

2 cups coconut flour

1 cup almond flour

2 tablespoons tapioca flour (or arrowroot powder)

2 eggs

1 tart apple

1 sweet apple

1/2 cup unsweetened applesauce

1/4 cup coconut oil

1/4 cup sweetener*

1 tablespoon baking soda

1 tablespoon apple cider vinegar

1 teaspoon ground cinnamon

1 teaspoon ground ginger

1 teaspoon sea salt

1/2 teaspoon ground white pepper (or ground black pepper)

INSTRUCTIONS

1. Preheat oven to 375 degrees F. Line 2 muffin pans with paper liners or coat with coconut oil.

2. Peel, core and grate or dice apples, and place in small bowl. Pour vinegar and spices over apples. Toss to coat.

3. In medium bowl, whisk eggs with hand mixer or whisk until light and thickened, about 2 minutes. Add applesauce, sweetener and coconut oil. Blend until combined. Mix in apples.

4. Sift flours, baking soda and salt into apple mixture and mix until combined.

5. Use ice cream scoop or tablespoon to scoop equal portions of batter into muffin pans until 2/3 - 3/4 full.

6. Place in oven and bake for 15 - 20 minutes, or until golden brown and firm but springy to the touch.

7. Remove form oven and let cool at least 5 minutes.

8. Serve warm/ Or allow to cool completely and serve room temperature.

NOTE: Bake in oiled square baking pan for 35 - 45 minutes or two loaf pans for 45 - 55 minutes for **Apple Bread Loaves**.

stevia, raw honey or agave nectar

Plain Pita

Prep Time: 5 minutes

Cook Time: 20 minutes

Servings: 1

INGREDIENTS

1 cup tapioca flour

1 cage-free egg

1/4 cup water

2 tablespoons coconut oil

1 teaspoon ground chia seed (or flax meal)

1/2 teaspoon baking soda

1/4 teaspoon ground white pepper (or black pepper)

1/4 teaspoon sea salt

INSTRUCTIONS

1. Preheat the oven to 375 degrees F. Line sheet pan with parchment paper or baking mat, or lightly coat with coconut oil. Heat small pot over low heat.

2. Add 1/3 cup tapioca flour, chia meal, water and 1 tablespoon coconut oil to pot. Stir until mixture comes together. Remove from heat and cool in freezer.

3. In medium bowl, blend remaining tapioca flour, baking soda, salt and pepper. Then add egg and remaining oil. Mix until combined.

4. Add cooled chia mixture to bowl. Mix to combine, then remove and knead briefly to bring together dough.

5. Form round disk, then flatten on prepared sheet pan to 1/4 - 1/3 inch with hands or rolling pin.

6. Place in oven and bake about 15 minutes. Carefully remove pan and turn pita over with spatula. Return to oven and bake another 5 - 10 minutes, or until crisp.

7. Remove from oven and fill with favorite Mediterranean meats. Or cut into wedges and dip into favorite spreads.

8. Serve warm or room temperature.

All-Purpose Pizza Crust

Prep Time: 5 minutes

Cook Time: 20 minutes

Servings: 2

INGREDIENTS

1/3 cup coconut flour

3 cage-free eggs

1/2 cup coconut milk

2 tablespoons flax meal (or ground chia seed)

2 tablespoons tapioca flour

1 teaspoon baking powder

1/2 teaspoon sea salt

INSTRUCTIONS

1. Preheat oven to 350 degrees F. Line sheet pan with parchment paper or baking mat, or coat lightly with coconut oil.
2. In medium bowl, beat eggs and coconut milk with hand mixer or whisk until well combined.
3. Sift coconut and tapioca flour, flax meal, baking powder and salt into egg mixture. Beat into thick batter.
4. Spread batter into desired shape on sheet pan with ladle or spatula.
5. Place in oven and bake for 10 minutes, or until firm enough to flip.
6. Carefully remove par baked crust. Peel away from sheet pan and turn over.

7. Return crust to oven and bake for additional 8 - 10 minutes, or until cooked through.

8. Remove crust and evenly spread with desired sauce and sprinkle with favorite toppings.

9. Set oven to broil. Broil pizza for 1 - 2 minutes, just to heat toppings.

10. Remove pizza and slice with knife or pizza cutter. Serve hot.

Strawberry Bread

Prep Time: 10 minutes

Cook Time: 10 minutes

Servings: 12 - 16

INGREDIENTS

1 cup coconut flour

3/4 cup cashew flour (or almond flour)

1/4 cup ground chia seed (or flax meal)

1/2 cup coconut oil

2 eggs

1/4 cup coconut crème

1/4 cup sweetener*

1/4 cup unsweetened apple sauce

1 teaspoons baking powder

1 tablespoon ground cinnamon

1 teaspoon ground ginger

1 teaspoon ground white pepper (or black pepper)

1 teaspoon sea salt

2 cups fresh sliced strawberries

1/2 cup chopped walnuts (optional)

INSTRUCTIONS

1. Preheat oven to 350 degrees F. Line muffin pan with paper liners or coat with coconut oil.

2. In large bowl, whisk eggs with hand mixer or whisk until frothy and light. Add coconut oil, sweetener and applesauce. Blend until combined. Slice strawberries, and fold in with walnuts (optional).

3. In medium bowl, blend flours, chia meal, baking powder, salt and spices. Stir flour blend into strawberry mixture until well combined.

4. Use ice cream scoop or tablespoon to scoop equal portions of batter into muffin pans, 1/2 - 3/4 full. Line or oil more muffin pans if excess batter remains.

5. Bake for 15 minutes, or until golden brown and firm but springy to the touch.

6. Cool enough to handle. Serve warm or room temperature.

NOTE: Bake in square oiled baking pan for 25 - 35 minutes or two oiled loaf pans for 35 - 45 minutes for **Strawberry Loaves**.

stevia, raw honey or agave nectar

Citrus Curry Spice Bread

Prep Time: 5 minutes

Cook Time: 20 minutes

Servings: 8

INGREDIENTS

2 cups almond flour

2 eggs

1/2 cup unsweetened applesauce

1/4 cup coconut oil

Juice of 1 lemon

Juice of 1 orange

1 teaspoon lemon zest

1 teaspoon orange zest

1 tablespoon apple cider vinegar

2 tablespoons baking powder

1 tablespoon vanilla

1 tablespoon curry powder

1 teaspoon ground cinnamon

1 teaspoon ground ginger

1 teaspoon ground white pepper (or black pepper)

1 teaspoon cardamom (optional)

1/ 4 cup pumpkin seeds (optional)

Pinch sea salt

INSTRUCTIONS

1. Preheat oven to 350 degrees F. Coat 2 small loaf pans with coconut oil.

2. Separate eggs. In large bowl, whisk egg whites to soft peaks with hand mixer or whisk. Add yolks, applesauce, oil, juices, zests and vinegar. Beat well.

3. In medium bowl, blend flour, baking powder, spices and salt. Stir flour mixture into egg mixture.

4. Pour batter into loaf pans and bake for 20 - 25 minutes, or until toothpick inserted into center comes out clean.

5. Let cool slightly. Insert knife around edges and remove from pan. Serve warm or room temperature.

NOTE: Bake in large oiled loaf pan for 35 - 45 minutes for **Citrus Curry Spice Loaf**.

stevia, raw honey or agave nectar

Cranberry Pistachio Scones

Prep Time: 10 minutes

Cook Time: 25 minutes

Servings: 8

INGREDIENTS

2 cups almond flour

1/3 cup arrowroot flour

1 egg

1/4 cup organic coconut oil

2 tablespoons liquid sweetener*

2 teaspoons baking powder

1/2 teaspoon vanilla

1/2 teaspoon sea salt

1/4 cup pistachio nuts

1/4 cup dried cranberries

INSTRUCTIONS

1. Preheat oven to 350 degrees F. Line sheet pan with parchment or coat with coconut oil.
2. Whisk together flours, baking powder, salt and vanilla in large mixing bowl.
3. In small mixing bowl, combine egg, oil and sweetener with hand mixer or whisk. Beat briskly while slowly pouring in coconut oil.
4. Add egg mixture to flour blend and mix until well combined.

5. Fold in cranberries and pistachios until incorporated. Form dough into ball and place on sheet pan . Pat down to flatten to about 1/2 inch thick circle.

6. Cut into eight wedges with pizza cutter or sharp knife. Arrange at least 1 inch apart on sheet pan and bake for 20 - 25 minutes , or until edges are golden brown.

7. Remove and cool. Serve room temperature.

fresh squeezed orange juice, raw honey, agave nectar or grade B maple syrup

Sweet Potato Basil Rolls

Prep Time: 10 minutes

Cook Time: 20 minutes

Servings: 6

INGREDIENTS

1 cup tapioca flour/starch

1/4 - 1/3 cup coconut flour

1 egg

1/3 cup warm water

1/4 cup coconut oil

1/2 cup organic canned yams

1 teaspoon baking soda

1 teaspoon apple cider vinegar

Medium bunch fresh basil leaves

1 teaspoon rosemary

1/2 teaspoon ground white pepper (or black pepper)

1 teaspoon sea salt

INSTRUCTIONS

1. Preheat oven to 350 degrees F. Line sheet pan with parchment paper or coat with coconut oil.
2. Whisk egg in small bowl. Chop basil and rosemary. Whisk yams, vinegar and herbs into egg.

3. In medium bowl, blend tapioca flour, 1/4 cup coconut flour, baking powder, salt and pepper. Stir in warm water and oil. Add sweet potato mixture and mix until well combined.

4. If necessary, add coconut flour or water 1 tablespoon at a time to form soft and slightly sticky dough.

5. Use ice cream scoop or large spoon to scoop out 6 portions of dough and roll into round or oblong balls. Dust hands with extra tapioca flour to prevent sticking.

6. Place rolls on sheet pan and pat down slightly. Bake 20 minutes, or until edges are golden brown and tops are firm. Serve warm or room temperature.

NOTE: For **Sweet Potato Basil French Bread**, roll dough into single log and bake at 325 degrees F for 30 - 35 minutes, or until outside is toasted and center is cooked through.

Low-Carb English Muffins

Prep Time: 5 minutes

Cook Time: 15 minutes

Servings: 4

INGREDIENTS

1/3 cup coconut flour

4 eggs

1/4 cup almond milk (or low-fat coconut milk)

2 tablespoons coconut oil

1 tablespoon unsweetened applesauce

1/2 teaspoon baking soda

1 teaspoon organic apple cider vinegar

Pinch sea salt

INSTRUCTIONS

1. Preheat oven to 400 degrees F. Coat 4 mini-round cake pans or 4-inch diameter oven safe ramekins with coconut oil.

2. In small mixing bowl mix baking soda and apple cider vinegar together. Set aside and allow to froth.

3. In medium bowl, beat eggs with hand mixer or whisk until thick and frothy. Add flour, milk, applesauce and salt. Combine.

4. Add baking soda and vinegar mixture and blend well until smooth and free of clumps.

5. Pour batter into pans or ramekins and bake for 12 - 15 minutes, until slightly golden and center is firm to the touch.

6. Remove muffins from oven. Loosen from sides of pan or container with knife turn out.

7. Serve warm. Muffins will have traditional **English Crumpet** texture.

NOTE: For crusty, American style **English Muffins**, cut in half and toast in skillet coated with coconut oil. Press muffin down in pan with spatula and flip, browning on both sides.

stevia, raw honey or agave nectar

Indian Naan

Prep Time: 5 minutes

Cook Time: 15 minutes

Servings: 4

INGREDIENTS

1/2 cup coconut flour

4 eggs

1/4 cup coconut oil

1/2 - 2/3 cup water

1/4 tsp baking powder

1/2 teaspoons sea salt

Coconut oil (for cooking)

INSTRUCTIONS

1. Heat medium skillet over medium-high heat and coat generously with coconut oil.
2. Blend flour, eggs, oil, baking powder, salt and 1/2 cup water in a food processor or bullet blender. Process until smooth. Add liquid if batter is too thick, and coconut flour if too thin. You want a moderately thin batter.
3. Pour 1/4th of batter into hot oiled skillet. Cook until naan bubbles and browns, about 2 minutes. Then flip and cook another 2 minutes, or until golden and firm.
4. Repeat with remaining batter. Re-oil pan as necessary.

5. Drain hot naan on paper towel. Serve warm.

NOTE: For softer **Baked Naan** , bake at 425 degrees F in two (2)9-inch round cake pans generously coated with coconut oil for 10 minutes, or until cooked through.

Soft Burger Buns

Prep Time: 5 minutes

Cook Time: 15 minutes

Servings: 6

INGREDIENTS

1/4 cup almond flour

1/4 cup coconut flour

4 eggs

2 tablespoons coconut oil

2 tablespoons unsweetened applesauce

1 teaspoon flax meal (or ground chia seed)

1 teaspoon baking powder

1/2 teaspoon sea salt

INSTRUCTIONS

1. Preheat oven to 350 degrees F. Line sheet pan with parchment paper, or lightly coat with coconut oil. Or lightly coat 6 mini round cake pans with coconut oil.

2. Beat eggs, coconut oil and applesauce in medium mixing bowl with hand mixer or whisk.

3. In large mixing bowl, sift together coconut flour, almond flour, flax or chia meal, baking powder and salt. Pour egg mixture into flour mixture and mix until combined.

4. Scoop thick batter onto prepared sheet pan in six 4 inch rounds. Or pour into six prepared mini cake pans for uniformity. Smooth batter with knife or spatula.
5. Place in oven and bake for 12 - 15 minutes, or until tops are firm to the touch and golden.
6. Remove from oven and let cool at least 5 minutes.
7. Slice in half and serve with your favorite patty or filling.

Sandwich Bread

Prep Time: 5 minutes

Cook Time: 15 minutes

Servings: 6

INGREDIENTS

2 cups almond flour

4 eggs

1/2 cup coconut cream (or melted cacao butter)

1/2 cup arrowroot powder (or tapioca flour)

1/3 cup ground chia seed (or flax meal)

1/4 cup coconut oil

2 tablespoons unsweetened applesauce

1 teaspoon apple cider vinegar

1 teaspoon baking soda

1/2 teaspoon sea salt

INSTRUCTIONS

1. Preheat oven to 350 degrees F. Lightly coat 6 mini round cake pans with coconut oil.

2. Beat eggs, coconut oil, coconut cream, applesauce and vinegar in medium mixing bowl with hand mixer or whisk.

3. In large mixing bowl, sift together almond flour, arrowroot, chia meal, baking soda and salt. Pour egg mixture into flour mixture and mix until well combined.

4. Pour batter into prepared mini cake pans and bake for about 15 minutes, or until golden brown and toothpick inserted comes out clean.
5. Remove from oven and let cool at least 5 minutes.
6. Slice in half and serve with your favorite deli meats or sandwich salads.

NOTE: Lightly oil medium loaf pan and bake for about 25 minutes for **Sandwich Bread** loaf.

Grain-Free Tortillas

Prep Time: 5 minutes

Cook Time: 10 minutes

Servings: 2

INGREDIENTS

2 tablespoons almond flour

2 tablespoons coconut flour

1/2 tablespoon flax meal (or ground chia seed)

2 eggs

1/4 cup water (plus extra)

2 tablespoons coconut oil

1/4 teaspoon baking powder

Coconut oil (for cooking)

INSTRUCTIONS

1. Heat medium frying pan over medium-high heat and coat with coconut oil.
2. Whisk together eggs, coconut oil and 1/4 cup water in medium bowl.
3. In separate mixing bowl, blend coconut flour, almond flour, flax or chia seed, and baking powder.
4. Slowly whisk as you pour flourmixture into wet ingredients. If batter appears too thick to spread fairly thin in pan, add up to 4 tablespoon water 1 tablespoon at a time.

5. Use ladle or dry measure cup to pour 1/2 of batter into hot oiled pan. Tilt pan in circular motion as you pour so batter spreads thinly.
6. Cook batter for about 2 minutes or until slightly golden and firm. Flip tortilla with tongs or spatula and cook another 2 minutes. Remove and place on paper towel or parchment.
7. Cook remaining batter for 2 minutes on each side. Re-oil pan as necessary.
8. Fill warm tortillas with meat or veggies of choice and serve warm.

Double Chocolate Chip Scone

Prep Time: 10 minutes

Cook Time: 25 minutes

Servings: 8

INGREDIENTS

2 cups almond flour

1/3 cup arrowroot flour

1 cage-free egg

1/4 cup coconut oil (or cacao or coconut butter, melted)

2 tablespoons raw honey (or agave)

2 tablespoons raw cocoa powder

2 teaspoons baking powder

1/2 teaspoon vanilla

1/2 teaspoon Celtic sea salt

1/2 cup organic chocolate chips (or chocolate bark or cacao nibs)

INSTRUCTIONS

1. Preheat oven to 350 degrees F. Line sheet pan with parchment or coat with coconut oil.
2. Whisk together almond flour, arrowroot flour, cocoa, baking powder, salt and vanilla in large mixing bowl.
3. In small mixing bowl, combine egg, and honey with hand mixer or whisk. Beat briskly while slowly pouring in oil or melted butter.
4. Add egg mixture to flour mixture blend and mix until well combined.

5. Roughly chop chocolate bark, if using. Fold in chocolate or cacao nibs until incorporated. Form dough into ball and place on sheet pan . Pat down to flatten to about 1/2 inch thick circle.

6. Cut into eight wedges with pizza cutter or sharp knife. Arrange at least 1 inch apart on prepared sheet pan.

7. Bake for 20 - 25 minutes , or until edges are browned.

8. Remove from oven and let cool completely.

9. Serve room temperature.

Pretzel Sticks

Prep Time: 15 minutes

Cook Time: 20 minutes

Servings: 12

INGREDIENTS

1 1/2 cups almond flour

3 tablespoons coconut flour

3 cage-free eggs

2 tablespoons ghee (or cacao butter or coconut oil, melted)

2 tablespoons Celtic sea salt

1 teaspoon water

INSTRUCTIONS

1. Beat 2 eggs in small mixing bowl with hand mixer to whisk. Set aside.

2. In medium bowl, sift almond flour, 1/2 teaspoon salt, and butter or oil. Mix to combine.

3. Add beaten eggs and 1 tablespoon coconut flour. Mix well. Let mixture sit 1 minute, then add second tablespoon of coconut flour. Blend again and let sit another minute. Add last tablespoon of coconut flour. Mix and set aside 5 minutes.

4. Preheat oven to 350 degrees F. Line sheet pan with parchment or baking mat.

5. Take portion of dough about the size of a golf ball and roll into long, thin log. Place on prepared sheet pan. Repeat with remaining dough.

6. Place pan in oven and bake 10 minutes.

7. Beat remaining egg in small bowl with 1 teaspoon water.

8. Remove pan from oven. Increase oven temperature to 400 degrees F.

9. Lightly brush tops of pretzels with the egg wash and sprinkle with generously with remaining salt.

10. Once oven is preheated, return pan to oven and bake 5 minutes.

11. Remove from oven and let cool slightly.

12. Serve warm. Or cool completely and serve room temperature.

Sweet Banana Shortbreads

Prep Time: 10 minutes

Cook Time: 30 minutes

Servings: 12

INGREDIENTS

1 cup coconut flour

2 overripe bananas

2 cage-free eggs

1/4 cup raw honey (or agave or date butter)

1/4 cup coconut oil (coconut or cacao butter)

1 teaspoon baking powder

1/2 teaspoon ground cinnamon

1/2 teaspoon vanilla

1/2 teaspoon of Celtic sea salt

INSTRUCTIONS

1. Preheat oven to 350 degrees F. Line sheet pan with baking mat or lightly coat with coconut oil.

2. Add eggs to food processor or high-speed blender and process until light and fluffy, about 2 minutes. Peel and add bananas, sweetener, oil or butter, cinnamon and vanilla. Process until well combined.

3. Add almond flour, baking powder and salt. Process until dough comes together.

4. Roll dough into 12 balls and place on prepared sheet pan. Press to flatten.

5. Bake 10 - 15 minutes, until golden around edges.

6. Remove from oven and allow to cool at least 5 minutes.

7. Serve warm. Or transfer to wire rack to cool completely and serve room temperature.

Lemon Lavender Scones

Prep Time: 10 minutes

Cook Time: 25 minutes

Servings: 8

INGREDIENTS

2 cups almond flour

1/3 cup arrowroot powder

1/4 cup coconut oil (or cacao or coconut butter, melted)

2 tablespoons raw honey (or agave or stevia)

1 cage-free egg

1 lemon

2 teaspoons baking powder

2 teaspoons crushed lavender buds (food-grade)

1/4 teaspoon vanilla

1/4 teaspoon Celtic sea salt

INSTRUCTIONS

1. Preheat oven to 350 degrees F. Line sheet pan with parchment or baking mat.
2. Whisk together almond flour, arrowroot, baking powder and salt in large mixing bowl. Add lavender.
3. Zest *then* juice lemon into small mixing bowl. Add egg, sweetener and vanilla and mix with hand mixer or whisk. Beat briskly while slowly pouring in oil or melted butter.

4. Pour egg mixture into flour mixture and mix until well combined, and dough comes together. Form dough into ball and place on prepared sheet pan. Flatten to about 1/2 inch thick circle.

5. Cut into eight wedges with pizza cutter or sharp knife. Arrange at least 1 inch apart on sheet pan and bake for 20 - 25 minutes, or until edges are browned.

6. Remove and let cool at least 10 minutes.

7. Serve warm. Or transfer to wire rack to cool completely and serve room temperature.

Indulgent Baked Treats

Strawberry Toaster Pastry

Prep Time: 25 minutes

Cook Time: 20 minutes

Servings: 4

INSTRUCTIONS

Crust

2 cups almond flour

2 cage-free eggs

1/4 cup coconut oil (or ghee, cacao butter or coconut butter, softened)

1 tablespoon date butter (or honey or agave)

1/4 teaspoon baking soda

1/4 teaspoon vanilla

1/2 teaspoon Celtic sea salt

Filling

2 cups chopped strawberries (about 3/4 pint whole strawberries) (fresh or frozen)

2 tablespoons raw honey (or agave)

1/2 teaspoon vanilla

1/4 teaspoon Celtic sea salt

INSTRUCTIONS

1. Preheat oven to 400 degrees. Line sheet pan with parchment or baking mat. Cover cutting board with parchment.

2. For *Crust*, sift almond flour into medium mixing bowl. Add baking soda, vanilla and salt.

3. In a small mixing bowl, whisk eggs and date butter. Add flour mixture and mix to combine. Add oil, ghee or butter and mix until malleable dough comes together.

4. Roll in plastic wrap or wrap tightly in parchment and refrigerate for 15 minutes.

5. Heat medium pan over medium heat.

6. Chop strawberries and add to hot pan with honey, vanilla and salt. Cook strawberries down until juices thicken and reduce, about 10 minutes. Stir occasionally.

7. Remove dough from refrigerator. Roll out dough on parchment covered cutting board to about 1/8 inch thick rectangle with rolling pin. Use sharp knife or pizza cutter to cut dough into 4 rectangles.

8. Scoop equal portions of *Filling* into center of one side of each dough rectangle. Fold bare half of dough over filled half. Press edges together, letting any trapped air escape. Crimp edges of dough together with fork. Repeat with remaining dough.

9. Arrange pastries on prepared sheet pan and bake 15 - 20 minutes, or until golden and cooked through.

10. Remove from oven and serve immediately. Or allow to cool and serve room temperature.

11. Reheat in toaster, if preferred.

Cocoa Zucchini Muffin

Prep Time: 10 minutes

Cook Time: 15 minutes

Servings: 12

INGREDIENTS

1 1/2 cups almond flour

2 cage-free eggs

1 small zucchini (about 1 cup grated)

1/2 cup unsweetened applesauce

1/4 cup date butter (or agave or raw honey)

1/4 cup coconut oil (or cacao or coconut butter, melted)

1/4 cup cocoa powder

2 tablespoons ground chia seed (or flax meal)

1 teaspoon baking soda

1 teaspoon baking powder

1 teaspoon vanilla

1 teaspoon ground cinnamon

1 teaspoon ground black pepper

1/2 teaspoon Celtic sea salt

1/4 cup cocoa nibs or chocolate chips (optional)

INSTRUCTIONS

1. Preheat oven to 350 degrees F. Line muffin pan with paper liners or lightly coat with coconut oil.

2. Add eggs, oil or melted butter, applesauce and date butter to food processor or high-speed blender. Process until thick, light mixture forms, about 1 - 2 minutes.

3. Sift almond flour, cocoa powder, chia or flax meal, baking soda and powder, salt and spices into processor. Process to combine, about 1 minute.

4. Grate zucchini and stir in with cocoa nibs or chocolate chips (optional).

5. Use scoop or tablespoon to pour batter into prepared muffin pan. Bake for about 15 - 20 minutes, until toothpick inserted into center comes out clean.

6. Remove from oven and let cool about 5 minutes.

7. Serve warm. Or let cool completely and serve room temperature.

Vanilla Bean Shortbread Cookies

Prep Time: 5 minutes

Cook Time: 20 minutes

Servings: 12

INGREDIENTS

1 2/3 cups almond flour

2/3 cup almonds (blanched, skinless)

1/4 cup coconut oil (or cacao butter or coconut butter, melted)

1/4 cup date butter (or raw honey or agave)

1 Madagascar whole vanilla bean

1/4 teaspoon baking soda

1/4 teaspoon Celtic sea salt (plus extra)

INSTRUCTIONS

1. Preheat oven to 300 degrees F. Line sheet pan with parchment or baking mat.
2. Add almonds to food processor or high-speed blender and process until finely ground, about 2 minutes.
3. Add ground almonds to medium mixing bowl. Sift in almond flour, baking soda and salt.
4. Split vanilla bean pod in half and scrap insides into small mixing bowl. Add oil or melted butter and date butter. Mix to combine.
5. Pour vanilla mixture into flour mixture and mix to form dough.

6. Use mini ice cream scoop or tablespoon to drop portions of dough onto prepared sheet pan. Bake for 20 minutes , or until lightly browned.

7. Remove from oven and let cool at least 5 minutes.

8. Serve warm. Or let cool completely and serve room temperature.

Cranberry Pistachio Biscotti

Prep Time: 15 minutes

Cook Time: 45 minutes*

Servings: 6

INGREDIENTS

1 cup almond flour

1/2 cup coconut flour

1/2 cup raw honey (or date butter or agave)

1/4 cup pistachios

1/4 cup dried cranberries

1/2 teaspoon vanilla

1/2 teaspoon baking soda

1/4 teaspoon Celtic sea salt

INSTRUCTIONS

1. Preheat oven to 350 degrees F. Line sheet pan with parchment paper. Heat medium pan over medium heat.

2. In medium mixing bowl, blend almond flour, coconut flour, baking soda and salt with hand mixer or whisk.

3. Beat in honey and vanilla until well combined and thick, sticky dough forms. Mix in pistachios and cranberries with wooden spoon.

4. Form dough into flattened, uniform mound about 1 inch thick on sheet pan. Pat down mound to keep any nuts from sticking out.

5. Bake for about 15 minutes. Remove from oven and allow to cool for about 15 minutes.

6. Use a very sharp serrated knife to carefully cut biscotti log into 1/2 - 2/3 inch slices. Hold on to the mound and cut on a diagonal. If it becomes crumbly, stick it back together.

7. Lay slices on their sides and return to oven for 15 minutes.

8. *Turn oven off and leave oven door open a crack. Allow biscotti to cool and dry for at least 2 hours.

9. Serve room temperature.

Skinny Cherry Pie

Prep Time: 30 minutes

Cook Time: 40 minutes

Servings: 12

INGREDIENTS

Crust

3 1/2 cups almond flour

2 cage-free eggs

1/2 cup coconut oil (or cacao butter or ghee)

1/2 cup nut milk (or water)

1/4 teaspoon Celtic sea salt

Filling

2 cups pitted cherries (fresh or frozen)

3/4 cup raw honey (or agave or date butter)

1/4 cup tapioca flour

1 tablespoon coconut oil (or cacao or coconut butter)

1/2 teaspoon vanilla

INSTRUCTIONS

1. *For *Crust*, blend almond flour and salt in small mixing bowl. Add eggs, oil or butter, and nut milk. Mix until dough forms, then divide. Roll half of dough into a round disc that will fit over pie pan, then cover with parchment paper. Press remaining dough into pie pan. Refrigerate dough for 30 minutes.

2. For *Filling*, add cherries, sweetener, coconut and vanilla to medium pot. Sift in tapioca and stir to combine. Heat pot over low heat and bring to simmer, about 10 - 15 minutes. Stir occasionally.

3. Once juice releases from cherries, increase heat to medium and bring to a boil, about 5 minutes. Stir frequently. Cook until juice reduces and mixture thickens, about 5 - 8 minutes. Remove from heat and set aside in refrigerator to cool.

4. Preheat oven to 375 degrees F.

5. Remove dough from refrigerator. Pour *Filling* into bottom *Crust*. Use pizza cutter or sharp knife to cut 1 inch strips from dough disc. Cover pie with dough strips in lattice (crisscross) formation. Press edges of dough together to create seal.

6. Bake about 40 minutes, until dough is golden brown and *Filling* is set.

7. Remove from oven and let cool about 20 minutes.

8. Slice and serve warm. Or let cool completely and serve room temperature.

Berry Cobbler

Prep Time: 5 minutes

Cook Time: 25 minutes

Servings: 8

INGREDIENTS

1 cup blueberries

1 cup raspberries

1 cup strawberries (chopped)

1 cup blackberries

2 tablespoons tapioca flour (or arrowroot powder)

1 teaspoon vanilla

1/2 teaspoon ground ginger

1/4 teaspoon Celtic sea salt

Crumble

1 cup almond flour

1/2 cup almonds

1/4 cup coconut oil (or cacao butter)

1/4 cup almond butter

1/4 cup dried pitted dates

1 teaspoon vanilla

1/2 teaspoon ground cinnamon

1/2 teaspoon Celtic sea salt

Raw honey (or agave or date butter) (optional)

INSTRUCTIONS

1. Preheat oven to 350 degrees F. Lightly coat sides of baking dish with coconut oil.

2. Add berries, vanilla, ginger and salt to medium mixing bowl. Sift tapioca into bowl and gently toss. Transfer to prepared baking dish and set aside.

3. For *Crumble*, add dates, oil or butter, and almonds to food processor or high-speed blender. Pulse until dates and almonds are finely chopped or coarsely ground.

4. Transfer to clean medium mixing bowl with almond flour, almond butter, vanilla, cinnamon and salt. Mix with hands or wooden spoon until crumbly mixture resembling moist graham cracker crust forms. Add sweetener to reach desired consistency, if necessary.

5. Sprinkle crumble evenly over berries and bake about 25 minutes, until crumble is golden brown and crisp.

6. Remove from oven and let cool about 5 minutes.

7. Serve warm. Or let cool completely and serve room temperature.

Vanilla Peach Cake

Prep Time: 10 minutes

Cook Time: 50 minutes

Servings: 12

INGREDIENTS

4 ripe peaches

3/4 cup coconut flour

10 cage-free eggs

1/2 cup coconut oil (or cacao or coconut butter)

1/3 cup raw honey (or agave, date butter or stevia)

2 tablespoons tapioca flour (or arrowroot powder)

1 teaspoon baking soda

1 1/2 teaspoons vanilla

1 teaspoon Celtic sea salt

INSTRUCTIONS

1. Preheat oven to 350 degrees F. Line square or rectangular baking dish with parchment paper, or coat with coconut oil.

2. Slice peaches in half, twist to release from pit and remove pit. Dice 2 peaches and set aside.

3. Roughly chop remaining peaches and add to food processor or high-speed blender. Process until almost smooth, about 1 minute.

4. Add eggs, oil or butter, and flour to processor in 2 batches. Process until well combined, about 1 - 2 minutes. Add sweetener, baking

soda, vanilla and salt. Process until light, thick batter forms. Stir in diced peaches.

5. Pour batter into prepared baking pan and bake about 50 minutes, until golden brown and toothpick inserted into center comes out moist but clean.

6. Remove from oven and let cool about 10 minutes.

7. Slice and serve warm. Or let cool completely and serve room temperature or warm.

Lemon Bundt Cake

Prep Time: 15 minutes

Cook Time: 45 minutes

Servings: 12

INGREDIENTS

6 cage-free eggs

1 cup almond flour

3 large lemons

1/2 cup raw honey (or agave or date butter)

1/4 cup coconut oil (cacao or coconut butter, melted)

2 teaspoons baking soda

1 teaspoon vanilla

1/2 teaspoon Celtic sea salt

INSTRUCTIONS

1. Preheat oven to 350 degrees F. Coat Bundt pan with coconut oil.
2. Add eggs to food processor or high-speed blender. Process until pale and lightened, about 2 minutes.
3. Zest 1 lemon, then juice all lemons into processor. Add flour, sweetener, oil or butter, baking soda, vanilla and salt. Process until well combined, about 1 - 2 minutes.
4. Pour batter into prepared Bundt pan and bake about 45 minutes, until golden brown and toothpick inserted halfway between center and edge of pan comes out clean.

5. Remove oven and let cool 15 minutes. Turn cake out onto serving dish.

6. Slice and serve warm. Or allow to cool completely and serve room temperature.

Chocolate Zucchini Cake

Prep Time: 10 minutes

Cook Time: 25 minutes

Servings: 12

INGREDIENTS

1 1/2 cups almond flour

2 cage-free eggs

1 medium zucchini (1 1/2 cups grated)

1/2 cup unsweetened applesauce

1/4 cup coconut oil

1/4 - 1/2 cup sweetener*

1/4 cup cocoa powder

2 tablespoons ground chia seed (or flax meal)

1 tcaspoon baking soda

1 teaspoon baking powder

1 teaspoon vanilla

1 teaspoon ground cinnamon

1 teaspoon ground black pepper

1/2 teaspoon sea salt

1/4 cup cocoa nibs or chocolate chips (optional)

INSTRUCTIONS

1. Preheat oven to 350 degrees F. Line rectangular baking pan with parchment or lightly coat with coconut oil.

2. Add eggs, coconut oil, applesauce and sweetener to food processor or bullet blender. Process until mixture is thick and lightened.

3. Grate zucchini and add to medium mixing bowl. Pour egg mixture over grated zucchini.

4. Sift almond flour, cocoa powder, chia meal, baking soda and powder, salt and spices into bowl. Beat with hand mixer or whisk to combine. Stir in cocoa nibs or chocolate chips (optional).

5. Pour batter into prepared baking pan and bake for about 25 minutes, until toothpick inserted into center comes out clean.

6. Remove from oven and let cool about 10 minutes.

7. Slice and serve warm. Or let cool completely and serve room temperature.

stevia, raw honey or agave nectar

Ginger Spice Cookies

Prep Time: 15 minutes

Cook Time: 15 minutes

Servings: 6

INGREDIENTS

1 1/2 cups almond flour

1 cage-free egg

1/4 cup sweetener*

2 tablespoons coconut oil

1 teaspoon ground chia seed (or flax meal)

1/4 teaspoon baking soda

1 tablespoon ground ginger

1/2 teaspoon ground clove

Pinch all spice

Pinch ground black pepper

Pinch sea salt

INSTRUCTIONS

1. Preheat oven to 350 degrees F. Line sheet pan with parchment or baking mat, or lightly coat with coconut oil.
2. Beat egg, oil, sweetener and chia meal in medium mixing bowl with hand mixer or whisk.
3. Add almond flour, baking soda, salt and spices. Mix until combined.
4. Chill batter in freezer for 5 - 10 minutes.

5. Scoop chilled batter into 6 large rounds on prepared sheet pan. Press into disk shape with hand.

6. Bake for about 15 minutes, until firm around the edges and golden brown.

7. Remove from oven and let cool about 10 minutes.

8. Serve warm. Or let cool completely and serve room temperature.

raw honey, agave nectar, grade B maple syrup, molasses

Orange Cranberry Muffins

Prep Time: 5 minutes

Cook Time: 20 minutes

Servings: 12

INGREDIENTS

1 1/2 cups almond flour

2 cage-free eggs

1/2 cup fresh squeezed orange juice (about 2 oranges)

1/4 cup coconut oil

1/4 cup dried cranberries

1 tablespoon orange zest

1 teaspoon baking powder

1/2 teaspoon vanilla

1/2 teaspoon sea salt

INSTRUCTIONS

1. Preheat oven to 350 degrees F. Line muffin pan with paper liners or coconut oil.

2. In medium bowl, beat eggs with hand mixer or whisk until light and a foamy. Add coconut oil, orange juice and zest. Beat well.

3. Sift in almond flour, baking powder, vanilla and salt. Mix until combined. Stir in cranberries.

4. Use ice cream scoop or tablespoon to scoop batter into prepared muffin pan.

5. Bake about 20 minutes, or until toothpick inserted into center comes out clean.
6. Remove from oven and serve warm. Or let cool completely and serve room temperature.

NOTE: Bake in oiled loaf pan for 40 - 45 minutes for **Cranberry Orange Bread**.

stevia, raw honey or agave nectar

Milano Cookie Sandwiches

Prep Time: 30 minutes

Cook Time: 15 minutes

Servings: 12

INGREDIENTS

Lady Fingers

1/3 cup coconut flour

3 tablespoons arrowroot powder

4 eggs

1/4 cup sweetener*

1/2 teaspoon baking powder

1/2 teaspoon vanilla

Chocolate Filling

4 oz organic dark chocolate

2 oz full-fat coconut milk

INSTRUCTIONS

1. Preheat oven to 400 degrees F. Line two sheet pans with parchment paper. Fit pastry bag with 1/2 inch round tip, or cut 1/4 inch corner off sturdy kitchen storage bag (like Ziploc®).
2. For *Lady Fingers*, beat egg yolks, sweetener and vanilla until thick and pale.
3. In separate bowl, beat egg whites to stiff peaks with hand mixer or whisk, about 8 minutes. Fold half of egg whites into egg yolk

mixture. Then sift in coconut flour, arrowroot powder and baking powder. Fold in remaining egg whites.

4. Scoop batter into pastry or storage bag. Place in tall wide contain and fold open end of bag over edge of container for easier prep.

5. Pipe 4 inch cookies onto prepared sheet pans about 2 inches apart.

6. Place in oven and bake for 8 minutes, until set and just golden.

7. Remove cookies from oven and transfer full parchment sheet onto wire rack to cool completely. Do not try to remove warm cookies from parchment.

8. Heat 1 inch water in bottom of double boiler, or in bottom pan with metal or class bowl on top.

9. For Chocolate Filling, melt chocolate and coconut milk over double boiler until smooth.

10. Remove cooled *Lady Fingers* from parchment. Dip bottom of cookie in melted chocolate and press against bottom of second cookie to make sandwich. Repeat with remaining cookies.

11. Serve warm. Let chocolate set for 10 minutes, in refrigerator if preferred, and serve chilled or room temperature.

stevia, raw honey or agave nectar

Cocoa Spice Pinwheel Cookies

Prep Time: 10 minutes

Cook Time: 20 minutes

Servings: 12

INGREDIENTS

2 cups almond flour

2 tablespoon sweetener*

1 egg

1 teaspoon vanilla

1/2 teaspoon baking powder

1/4 teaspoon sea salt

Filling

2 tablespoons cocoa powder

2 tablespoons sweetener*

2 teaspoons ground cinnamon

1 teaspoon ground black pepper

1/2 teaspoon vanilla

INSTRUCTIONS

1. Preheat oven to 300 degrees F. Line sheet pan with parchment or baking mat. Prepare 2 additional sheets of parchment.

2. Add flour, egg, sweetener, vanilla, baking powder and salt to medium bowl. Blend with wooden spoon, then knead with hand to form thick dough.

3. Divide dough in half. Place half of dough in small mixing bowl. Add all *Filling* ingredients to bowl and mix until well combined.

4. Roll out each half of dough separately on parchment sheets. Roll into equal rectangles.

5. Place *Filling* rectangle on top of plain dough. Use parchment to help roll dough tightly along long edge into log.

6. Use sharp knife to cut log into 1/4 round slices. Place cookies on prepared sheet pan and bake about 10 minutes, until edges are golden brown.

7. Remove from oven and let cool about 5 minutes.

8. Serve warm. Or let cool completely and serve room temperature.

*raw honey, agave nectar or maple syrup

Skinny Key Lime Coconut Bars

Prep Time: 15 minutes

Cook Time: 30 minutes

Servings: 12

INGREDIENTS

Crust

1/2 cup raw cashews

2/3 cup coconut flour

2 eggs

2 tablespoons coconut oil

2 tablespoons sweetener*

1 tablespoon flaked or shredded coconut

1 teaspoon fresh lime juice

1/2 teaspoon baking soda

1/2 teaspoon vanilla

Filling

2 eggs

2 egg yolks

1 cup fresh key lime juice or (about 12 key limes - sub 10 Persian limes)

1/2 cup sweetener*

1/3 - 1/2 cup flaked or shredded coconut

2 tablespoons coconut flour

1 teaspoon lime zest

INSTRUCTIONS

1. Preheat oven to 350 degrees F. Lightly coat rectangular baking dish with coconut oil, or line with parchment.

2. For *Crust*, add cashews and coconut to food processor or bullet blender and process until finely ground. Add remaining *Crust* ingredients to food processor and pulse until dough comes together.

3. Press dough into bottom of baking dish, and slightly up the sides. Dock crust with fork to prevent bubbling.

4. Place crust in oven and bake for 8 - 10 minutes.

5. For *Filling*, beat together eggs, egg yolks, lime juice, lime zest and sweetener with hand mixer or whisk in medium bowl.

6. Sift in coconut flour and beat to combine. Let mixture sit for 5 minutes. Add coconut and beat again.

7. Pour *Filling* over par baked crust. Place in oven and bake 20 minutes, until center is set but still jiggles slightly.

8. Remove from oven and let cool for 20 minutes. Refrigerate about 20 minutes, until fully set and chilled.

9. Serve chilled or room temperature.

raw honey or agave nectar

Coconut Baked Donut

Prep Time: 5 minutes

Cook Time: 20 minutes

Servings: 6

INGREDIENTS

Donuts

1 3/4 cups almond flour

1 tablespoon coconut flour

2 eggs

1/3 cup coconut oil

1/4 cup unsweetened applesauce

1/4 cup sweetener*

2 tablespoons nut milk

2 teaspoons vanilla

3/4 teaspoon baking soda

1/2 teaspoon sea salt

Topping

1/2 cup flaked or shredded coconut

1/4 cup full-fat coconut milk

2 tablespoon sweetener

1/4 teaspoon vanilla

INSTRUCTIONS

1. Preheat oven to 350 degrees F. Lightly coat donut pan with coconut oil.

2. Add almond and coconut flours, baking soda and salt to food processor or high-speed blender. Process for 1 minute.

3. Add eggs, sweetener, coconut oil, applesauce, nut milk and vanilla. Process until light, thick batter forms, about 1 - 2 minutes.

4. Pour batter into donut pan until wells are 3/4 full.

5. Place in oven and bake for about 20 minutes, until dough is set and lightly browned.

6. For *Topping*, combine coconut milk, sweetener and vanilla in small mixing bowl.

7. Remove pan from oven at let cool about 5 minutes. Then remove donuts from pan.

8. Dip donuts in coconut icing then sprinkle with flaked or shredded coconut.

9. Transfer decorated donuts to serving dish.

10. Serve warm. Or let cool completely and serve room temperature.

NOTE: Bake in 8 mini cake pans or specialty cake pop pans lightly coated with coconut oil for fillable donuts or donut holes if you do not have a donut pan.

* *stevia, raw honey or agave nectar*

Soft Pumpkin Cookies

Prep Time: 15 minutes

Cook Time: 20 minutes

Servings: 15

INGREDIENTS

Sweet Potato Cookies

1 cup almond flour

3/4 cup organic pumpkin purée

1/4 cup full-fat coconut milk

1 egg

1 orange

2 tablespoons sweetener*

1/2 teaspoon baking powder

1 teaspoon ground cinnamon

1/4 teaspoon ground ginger

1/4 teaspoon ground nutmeg

1/4 teaspoon ground white pepper (or ground black pepper)

INSTRUCTIONS

1. Preheat oven to 400 degrees F. Line sheet pan with parchment or lightly coat with coconut oil.
2. Zest *then* juice orange into medium mixing bowl. Beat in egg, coconut milk and sweetener with hand mixer or whisk.
3. Sift flour, baking powder and spices into bowl and mix well. Add pumpkin purée and mix to combine.

4. Scoop 15 cookies onto prepared sheet pan. Place in oven for about 20 minutes, until golden and set.
5. Remove and serve warm. Or allow to cool completely and serve room temperature.

raw honey, agave nectar or maple syrup

Asian Orange Muffins

Prep Time: 10 minutes

Cook Time: 15 minutes

Servings: 12

INGREDIENTS

1 1/2 cups almond flour

2 eggs

1 1/2 cups grated carrot

1/4 cup coconut oil

1/4 cup unsweetened applesauce

1/2 cup fresh squeezed orange juice

1 tablespoon orange zest

1 tablespoon grated fresh ginger

1 tablespoon ground ginger

1 teaspoon vanilla

1 teaspoon baking soda

1 teaspoon baking powder

1/2 teaspoon sea salt

INSTRUCTIONS

1. Preheat oven to 350 degrees F. Line muffin pan with paper liners or coconut oil.

2. Peel ginger. Grate ginger and carrots. In medium bowl beat eggs with hand mixer or whisk until light and a bit frothy. Add oil,

applesauce, orange juice and zest. Beat well. Fold in carrots and ginger.

3. Sift and stir in flour, baking soda and powder, spices and salt until combined.

4. Use ice cream scoop or tablespoon to scoop batter into muffin tins, about 1/2 - 3/4 full.

5. Bake 15 - 18 minutes, or until toothpick inserted into center comes out clean.

6. Serve warm or room temperature.

NOTE: Bake in oiled loaf pan for 35 - 45 minutes for **Asian Orange Bread**.

stevia, raw honey or agave nectar

Coconut Crisps

Prep Time: 10 minutes

Cook Time: 10 minutes

Servings: 4

INGREDIENTS

1 cup coconut flour

3/4 cup almond flour

4 egg whites

1/4 cup coconut oil

1/4 cup coconut crème

1/4 cup sweetener

1/2 cup flaked coconut

1 teaspoon vanilla

1/2 teaspoon baking soda

3/4 teaspoon sea salt

1/2 teaspoon ground white pepper (or black pepper)

INSTRUCTIONS

1. Preheat oven to 375 degrees F. Line sheet pan with parchment paper or coat with coconut oil. Prepare two additional sheets of parchment.

2. Whisk egg and oil with hand mixer or whisk until blended and slightly frothy. Add sweetener, coconut crème and vanilla, and continue blending.

3. Sift in half of flour, baking soda, vanilla, salt and pepper. Add coconut flakes. Sift in remaining flour. Stir and bring dough together.

4. Form dough into rectangle and flatten with hands on parchment. Cover with second sheet of parchment and flatten to about 1/4 inch with rolling pin. Remove top layer of parchment.

5. Cut rectangles from dough with pizza cutter or sharp knife. Carefully flip dough onto sheet pan. Arrange at least 1/2 inch apart on sheet pan.

6. Bake for about 10 minutes, or until crisp and golden brown. Remove and let cool. Serve room temperature.

Pecan Chess Pies

Prep Time: 20 minutes

Cook Time: 25 minutes

Servings: 6

INGREDIENTS

Crust

1 1/2 cups almond flour

1/2 cup pecans

1 egg

2 tablespoons coconut oil

1/4 teaspoon sea salt

Filling

1 cup full-fat coconut milk

2 cups pecans

1 cup dried pitted dates

1/2 cup sweetener*

2 eggs

2 egg yolks

1 1/2 tablespoons arrowroot powder

2 tablespoons coconut oil

1 teaspoon vanilla

INSTRUCTIONS

1. Preheat oven to 350 degrees F. Coat 6 mini pie plates or pie pans with coconut oil. Bring small pot of water to boil, leaving room for dates.

2. Add dates to boiling water for about 5 - 10 minutes, until tender. Then drain.

3. For *Crust*, process pecans in food processor or bullet lender until well ground. Add to small mixing bowl with almond flour and salt. Mix in oil and egg until dough forms.

4. Press dough into pie plates with hand or wooden spoon. Bake about 10 minutes, until golden. Remove pie shells from oven and set aside.

5. Chop 1 cup pecans and set aside

6. For *Filling*, process softened dates in food processor or bullet blender with about half of coconut milk. Add to medium mixing bowl with remaining coconut milk, sweetener, eggs, egg yolks, coconut oil, vanilla and arrowroot powder. Beat with hand mixer or whisk until combined and a bit airy. Mix in chopped pecans.

7. Pour batter into mini pie crusts. Top with whole pecans and bake for 20 - 25 minutes, until filling is set.

8. Remove pies and let cool about 20 minutes before serving.

9. Serve warm. Or refrigerate and serve cold. Also great at room temperature.

stevia, raw honey or agave nectar

NOTE: For large **Pecan Chess Pie**, bake in 9-inch pie plate for 45 - 55 minutes, or until center is set.

Mixed Berry Trifle

Prep Time: 10 minutes

Cook Time: 25 minutes

Servings: 12

INGREDIENTS

Cake

1 cup almond flour

1 cup coconut flour

3/4 cup coconut milk

4 eggs

1/2 cup sweetener*

1/2 cup coconut oil

2 tablespoons vanilla

2 teaspoons baking soda

Filling

1 cup coconut cream

2 tablespoons sweetener*

1 cup strawberries

1/2 cup blueberries

1/2 cup raspberries

1/2 cup blackberries

Juice of orange half

Juice of lemon half

Zest of orange half

Zest of lemon half

1/4 cup pistachios

INSTRUCTIONS

1. Preheat oven to 350 degrees F. Line muffin pan with paper liner or coat with coconut oil.
2. In large mixing bowl, beat eggs and coconut milk until light and airy. Beat in sweetener, oil and vanilla.
3. Sift in almond flour, coconut flour and baking soda. Mix until well combined.
4. Use ice cream scoop or spoon to scoop batter into muffin pan. Fill each cup 1/2 - 2/3 full with batter.
5. Bake in for about 15 minutes, until firm but springy in the center.
6. Remove cupcakes from oven and turn out onto wire rack or plate. Allow to cool for about 10 minutes and remove paper liners.
7. Dice strawberries and add to medium bowl with blueberries, raspberries, blackberries, lemon and orange zests and juices. Toss to combine.
8. In small bowl, mixi coconut cream with 2 tablespoon sweetener.
9. Slice cupcake in half to create top and bottom. Dollop coconut cream onto bottom half, then top with a spoonful of fruit. Drain juice from spoon before adding to cake.
10. Place cupcake top on top of fruit. Press down slightly. Add another dollop of coconut cream and another spoonful of fruit. Repeat with remaining cupcakes.
11. Serve room temperature. Or chill for 30 minutes and serve.

NOTE: Bake cake in 3 round cake pans for 20 minutes, then layer with cream and berries and stack for **Mixed Berry Trifle Cake**.

stevia, raw honey or agave nectar

Sugar Cookies

Prep Time: 10 minutes

Cook Time: 15 minutes

Servings: 12

INGREDIENTS

1 1/2 cups almond flour

1 cup coconut flour

1/2 cup sweetener*

5 dried pitted dates

1 egg

2 teaspoons coconut oil

1 teaspoon vanilla

1/2 teaspoon baking soda

Pinch sea salt

Water

INSTRUCTIONS

1. Preheat oven to 350 degrees F. Line sheet pan with parchment paper. Bring small pot of water to boil. Add dates and boil for about 5 - 8 minutes, until softened.

2. Add dates to food processor or bullet blender and process until smooth. Add leftover water if necessary.

3. Add sweetener, egg, oil and vanilla to dates and process until smooth.

4. Add date mixture to medium bowl. Sift in almond flour, coconut flour baking soda and salt. Beat with hand mixer until combined and smooth, about 5 minutes.

5. Roll dough into a log about 3 inches in diameter. Slice into 1/4 inch thick disks.

6. Place disks on sheet pan and bake for about 8 - 10 minutes.

7. Remove form oven and cool for a few minutes.

8. Serve warm or room temperature.

*stevia, raw honey or agave nectar

Apple Dump Muffins

Prep Time: 15 minutes

Cook Time: 25 minutes

Servings: 12

INGREDIENTS

6 medium apples

1 cup almond flour

1/4 cup tapioca flour

3 eggs

1/2 cup coconut oil

1/2 cup sweetener*

2 teaspoons baking powder

2 tablespoons ground cinnamon

1 teaspoon ground nutmeg

1 teaspoon sea salt

1/2 teaspoon black pepper (or white pepper)

Juice of lemon half

INSTRUCTIONS

1. Preheat oven to 350 degrees F. Lightly coat muffin pan with coconut oil, or line with paper liners.

2. Peel, core and thinly slice apples. Add to medium bowl with 1 tablespoon cinnamon and juice of half a lemon. Evenly sprinkle on tapioca flour and carefully toss with hands to coat apples.

3. In medium mixing bowl, blend almond flour, baking powder, spices and salt. Beat in eggs, sweetener and coconut oil with hand mixer or whisk. Fold in sliced apples.

4. Scoop batter into muffin pan and bake for 20 -25 minutes, or until top is browned and firm but springy. A toothpick inserted into the center should come our moist but clean.

5. Serve warm solo, or drizzled with your favorite sweetener.

NOTE: For *Apple Dump Cake*, bake in square baking dish or Bundt pan for 40 - 50 minutes.

raw honey, agave nectar or maple syrup

Fruit And Nut Cake

Prep Time: 10 minutes

Cook Time: 25 minutes

Servings: 8

INGREDIENTS

1 1/2 cup almond flour

4 eggs

2 tablespoons coconut oil

Juice of orange half

1/4 cup sweetener*

1/2 cup walnuts

1/4 cup pecans

1/2 cup dried pitted dates

1/2 cup dried cherries

1/4 cup dried apricots

1/4 cup raisins

1/2 teaspoon baking soda

1 teaspoon ground ginger

1 teaspoon vanilla

1/2 teaspoon sea salt

Zest of orange half

INSTRUCTIONS

1. Preheat oven to 350 degrees F. Lightly coat 2 small loaf pans or one Bundt pan with coconut oil.

2. Sift almond flour, baking soda and salt into large mixing bowl.

3. Chop walnuts, pecans, apricots and dates. Then stir all dried fruit and nuts into flour mixture.

4. In medium mixing bowl, mix eggs, coconut oil, juice and zest of half an orange, sweetener, ginger and vanilla. Then pour and mix into dry ingredients until just combined.

5. Scoop batter into loaf pans or Bundt pan, and smooth tops with spatula.

6. Bake 20 - 30 minutes, or until firm, browned and firm in the center.

7. Remove from oven and allow to cool before slicing.

8. Serve warm or room temperature.

*stevia, raw honey or agave nectar

Honey Nut Bun

Prep Time: 15 minutes

Cook Time: 30 minutes

Servings: 4

INGREDIENTS

Bun

1 cup tapioca flour/starch

1/4 - 1/3 cup coconut flour

1 egg

1/2 cup warm water

1/2 cup coconut oil

1 teaspoon apple cider vinegar

1 teaspoon vanilla

1/2 teaspoon cinnamon

1/2 teaspoon baking soda

1/2 teaspoon sea salt

Filling

1 cup walnuts

1/4 cup sweetener*

2 teaspoons cinnamon

1 teaspoon ground ginger

INSTRUCTIONS

1. Preheat oven to 350 degrees F. Line sheet pan with parchment paper or coat with coconut oil. Heat medium skillet over medium-high heat.

2. For *Filling*, mix walnuts, sweetener, cinnamon and ginger in small mixing bowl. Set aside.

3. In medium bowl, sift together tapioca flour, 1/4 cup coconut flour, vanilla, cinnamon, baking soda and salt. Stir in warm water and oil.

4. Whisk egg and vinegar in small bowl. Add egg mixture to flour mixture and mix until well combined.

5. Add 1 tablespoon coconut flour or water at a time if needed to form soft and slightly sticky dough.

6. Divide dough into 4 portions and flatten into round disks. Dust your hand or rolling pin with extra tapioca flour to prevent sticking.

7. Scoop *Filling* into center of dough disks and pinch edges of dough together to create round, sealed ball.

8. Place buns sealed side down on sheet pan and pat down slightly. Bake 20 minutes, or until edges are golden brown and dough is cooked through.

9. Serve immediately. Or store in lidded container.

*stevia, raw honey or agave nectar

Orange Anzac Biscuits

Prep Time: 5 minutes

Cook Time: 25 minutes

Servings: 12

INGREDIENTS

3/4 cup almond flour

3/4 cup sliced almonds

3/4 cup flaked or shredded coconut

1/4 cup date butter (raw honey or agave)

1/4 cup coconut oil (or ghee or cacao butter, melted)

1 orange (or tangerine or Clementine)

1/2 teaspoon baking soda

1/4 teaspoon ground ginger

INSTRUCTIONS

1. Preheat oven to 300 degrees F. Line sheet pan with parchment sheet or baking mat.

2. In medium mixing bowl, combine almond flour, sliced almonds and coconut.

3. Zest *then* juice orange into small mixings bowl. Add date butter and oil or melted butter. Mix to combine.

4. Add wet mixture to dry mixture and mix until dough comes together.

5. Form 12 large biscuits with tablespoon or scoop. Place on prepared sheet pan and flatten slightly.

6. Bake for 25 - 30 minutes, until golden. Remove from oven and let cool slightly before serving.

7. Serve warm. Or allow to cool completely and store in airtight container.

Sweet Cherry Fig Newtons

Prep Time: 10 minutes

Cook Time: 15 minutes

Servings: 12

INSTRUCTIONS

Cookie Dough

1 1/2 cups almond flour

1/4 cup dried pitted dates

1/4 cup date butter (or agave or honey)

1/4 cup coconut oil (or cacao or coconut butter, melted)

1 teaspoon vanilla

1/4 teaspoon Celtic sea salt

Cherry Fig Filling

1/2 cup dried black mission figs

1/4 cup pitted cherries (fresh or thawed)

1/4 teaspoon ground ginger

INSTRUCTIONS

1. Preheat oven to 350 degrees F. Line sheet pan with parchment or baking mat.
2. For *Cookie Dough*, Add dried dates, date butter, and oil or melted butter to food processor or high-speed blender. Process until coarsely ground, about 1 - 2 minutes.

3. Sift almond flour and salt into medium mixing bowl. Add date mixture to flour mixture and mix to combine. Set aside.

4. For *Filling*, remove stems from figs and add to clean food processor or high-speed blender with cherries and ginger. Process until smooth mixture forms, about 2 minutes. Set aside.

5. Divide dough in half. Roll first half of dough into long, thin rectangle about 1/4 inch thick between 2 parchment sheets.

6. Spread 1/2 of *Cherry Fig Filling* along one side of the dough, long-ways.

7. Use parchment to fold dough in half along long edge so plain dough covers side with *Cherry Fig Filling*. Dough should resemble flattened log.

8. Press edges of dough together for tight seal. Place on prepared sheet pan. Repeat with remaining *Cookie Dough* and *Cherry Fig Filling*.

9. Bake for 12 - 15 minutes, or until the edges are golden brown.

10. Remove from the oven and let cool about 5 minutes. Then slice logs into 2 inch cookies.

11. Serve immediately. Or allow to cool completely and serve room temperature.

Pineapple Upside Down Cake

Prep Time: 20 minutes

Cook Time: 4 hours

Servings: 8

INGREDIENTS

1 can (20 oz) organic pineapple rings (in juice)

2 cage-free eggs

1 cup almond flour

1/4 cup coconut flour

2 tablespoons tapioca flour (or arrow root powder)

1/2 cup coconut milk (optional)

1/4 cup coconut oil

1/4 cup date butter (or raw honey or agave)

3 tablespoons cacao butter (or coconut butter, softened)

1/2 teaspoon baking soda

1/2 teaspoon baking powder

1 teaspoon vanilla

1/4 teaspoon Celtic sea salt

INSTRUCTIONS

1. Spread softened butter over bottom of slow cooker. Then spread date butter over bottom of slow cooker. Place pineapple slices in bottom of slow cooker.

2. Place remaining pineapple and juice into food processor or high-speed blender. Process until smooth, about 30 seconds.

3. Add eggs, coconut oil, almond flour, coconut flour, tapioca flour, baking soda, baking powder, vanilla and salt to processor. Process until smooth batter forms, about 1 - 2 minutes.

4. Spoon batter into pineapple, filling in any gaps between fruit and slow cooker bottom.

5. Cover slow cooker with tea towel, then with lid. Turn on to high and cook 45 minutes. Decrease temperature to low and cook 3 - 4 hours, until cooked through but still moist.

6. Turn off slow cooker and carefully remove lid. Carefully remove slow cooker dish let cool at least 20 minutes.

7. Invert cake onto serving dish. Slice and serve warm.

8. Or let cool completely and serve room temperature.

Simple Chinese Moon Cakes

Prep Time: 5 minutes*

Cook Time: 15 minutes

Servings: 12

INGREDIENTS

2/3 cup coconut flour

2 cage-free egg yolks

1/2 cup ghee (or cacao or coconut butter)

1/4 cup date butter (or agave or raw honey)

Filling

1 cup dried fruit (apricots, strawberries, blueberries, etc.)

Water

INSTRUCTIONS

1. Preheat oven to 375 degrees F. Cover sheet pan with parchment or baking mat.

2. In medium mixing bowl, cream ghee, sweetener and 1 egg yolk with hand mixer or wooden spoon. Add flour and mix until dough comes together.

3. *Wrap dough in plastic wrap or parchment and refrigerate 30 minutes.

4. For *Filling*, add dried apricots to clean food processor or high-speed blender. Process until thick jam forms, about 1 - 2 minutes. Add enough water to reach desired consistency.

5. Remove dough from refrigerator. Form 24 balls from dough and place on prepared sheet pan. Press thumb into each ball to create indent.

6. Fill each indent with *Filling*. Add remaining egg yolk and 1 teaspoon water to small mixing bowl and brush each *Moon Cake* with egg wash.

7. Bake 15 - 20 minutes, until edges are slightly browned.

8. Remove from oven and let cool about 5 minutes.

9. Serve warm. Or transfer to wire rack to cool completely and serve room temperature.

Walnut Raisin Cookies

Prep Time: 10 minutes

Cook Time: 15 minutes

Servings: 12

INGREDIENTS

1 1/4 cups almond flour

1 cage-free egg

1/4 cup coconut oil (or cacao or coconut butter)

1/4 cup raw honey (or agave or date butter)

1/4 cup cashew butter

1/2 cup walnuts

1/4 cup raisins

1 teaspoon baking powder

1 teaspoon vanilla

1/4 teaspoon Celtic sea salt

INSTRUCTIONS

1. Preheat oven to 350 degrees F. Line sheet pan with parchment or baking mat.
2. Sift flour, baking powder and salt into medium mixing bowl. Beat with whisk or hand mixer to lighten. Add egg, oil or butter, sweetener, cashew butter, vanilla and salt. Mix well to form dough.
3. Chop walnuts and add to bowl with raisins. Mix to combine.

4. Shape dough into 12 balls and place onto prepared baking sheet. Flatten slightly with hand or spatula.

5. Place in oven and bake 10 - 15 minutes, until golden brown along edges.

6. Remove from oven and let cool 5 minutes.

7. Serve warm. Or transfer to wire rack to cool completely and serve room temperature.

Apple Upside Down Cakes

Prep Time: 5 minutes

Cook Time: 15 minutes

Servings: 2

INGREDIENTS

1 3/4 cups almond meal

2 eggs

3/4 cup almond milk

2 tablespoons sweetener*

1 teaspoon baking powder

Juice of 1/2 lemon

1 teaspoon vanilla

1 teaspoon ground cinnamon

1 teaspoon ground nutmeg

1/4 teaspoon salt

1 tart apple

1/2 cup crushed pecans

INSTRUCTIONS

1. Heat large skillet over medium-high heat and lightly coat with coconut oil.

2. In medium bowl combine lemon juice, vanilla, cinnamon and nutmeg.

3. Peel and core apple, then slice in half length-wise. Lay halves down on flat side and slice thinly from top of apple to bottom.

Carefully toss apple slices in lemon juice and spices. Try not to break any.

4. Arrange apple slices into a circle by overlapping at the bottom and fanning out. Try to make at least 4 circles.
5. Add eggs and almond milk into leftover lemon juice and spices and whisk until combined. Add almond flour, salt and baking powder. Whisk until smooth.
6. Use oiled spatula to lift apples, keeping their arrangement, and place into hot pan. Get at least two apple arrangements into pan together. Sprinkle chopped pecans into pan around apple circles.
7. Use ladle or dry measure cup to pour 1/3 cup of batter over and around apple arrangements in skillet. Do not let pancakes touch as they spread.
8. Cook until sides of pancakes are firm and batter bubbles up a bit. About 3 - 4 minutes.
9. Flip pancakes with spatula, careful not to disturb apples. Cook for additional minute, or until cooked through. Repeat with remaining batter. Re-oil pan if necessary.
10. Pancakes will be slightly delicate, so flip and plate with care.
11. Sprinkle with cinnamon. Serve warm.

stevia, raw honey, or agave nectar

Guilt Free Desserts

Skinny Apple Crumble

Prep Time: 20 minutes

Cook Time: 50 minutes

Servings: 8

INGREDIENTS

Crust

2 cups almond flour

1 cage-free egg

2 tablespoons coconut oil (or cacao butter or ghee)

1/4 teaspoon Celtic sea salt

Filling

5 apples

1/2 cup date butter (or raw honey or agave)

1/2 lemon

1 teaspoon ground cinnamon

1/2 teaspoon vanilla

1/4 teaspoon ground nutmeg

1/4 teaspoon Celtic sea salt

Topping

1/2 cup almond flour

1/2 cup pecans

1/2 cup shredded coconut

1/4 cup cold cacao butter (or coconut butter, ghee or coconut oil)

1/4 cup raw honey (or agave)

1/4 cup dried pitted dates

2 tablespoons ground flax

1 teaspoon cinnamon

INSTRUCTIONS

1. Preheat oven to 375 degrees F.
2. For *Crust*, blend almond flour and salt in small mixing bowl. Add egg and oil or butter. Mix until dough forms. Press into pie pan or baking dish with hand or wooden spoon. Set aside.
3. For *Filling*, core and peel apples. Cut into thin slices and add to large mixing bowl. Add sweetener, salt and spices. Juice 1/2 lemon over apples and mix to combine. Press apples firmly into *Crust*.
4. For *Topping*, add dates and honey or agave to food processor or high-speed blender. Process until coarsely ground, about 1 minute. Add butter or oil, almond flour, pecans, coconut, flax and cinnamon. Pulse until finely chopped or coarsely ground. Sprinkle *Topping* over apples.
5. Bake 40 - 50 minutes, until apples are cooked and *Topping* is browned and crisp.
6. Remove from oven and allow to cool at least 5 minutes.
7. Slice and serve warm. Or let cool completed and serve room temperature.

Creamy Pumpkin Cheesecake

Prep Time: 15 minutes*

Cook Time: 10 Minutes

Servings: 12

INGREDIENTS

Crust

1/2 cup coconut flour

1/4 cup cacao butter (or coconut butter or coconut oil)

1/4 cup raw honey (or agave or date butter)

1/2 cup shredded or flaked coconut

Filling

1 1/2 cups raw cashews

1 cup organic pumpkin purée

1/2 cup date butter (or agave or raw honey)

1/2 cup full-fat coconut milk

1/2 cup coconut oil (or cacao or coconut butter, melted)

1 lemon

1 1/2 teaspoons vanilla

2 teaspoons ground cinnamon

1/2 teaspoon ground nutmeg

1/4 teaspoon ground clove

1/4 teaspoon ground ginger

1/2 teaspoon Celtic sea salt

Water

INSTRUCTIONS

1. *For *Filling*, soak cashews in enough water to cover for at least 4 hours to overnight in refrigerator. Drain and rinse.

2. Preheat oven to 375 degrees F.

3. For *Crust*, place all ingredients in food processor or high-speed blender. Process until well ground and mixture sticks together, about 2 minutes.

4. Press *Crust* firmly into bottom of spring form pan with hands. Bake about 8 minutes, then set aside.

5. For *Filling*, zest *then* juice lemon into clean food processor or high-speed blender. Add soaked cashews, pumpkin purée, sweetener, coconut milk, oil or butter, vanilla, salt and spices. Process until smooth, about 2 - 3 minutes.

6. Pour *Filling* into *Crust* and smooth with spatula.

7. *Cover pie with parchment, if preferred, and set aside in refrigerator at least 4 hours to set.

8. Slice and serve chilled.

Gingerbread Cookies

Prep Time: 5 minutes

Cook Time: 15 minutes

Servings: 12

INGREDIENTS

1 cup almond flour

2 cage-free eggs

1/2 cup dried pitted dates

1/4 cup raw honey (or dark agave)

1/4 cup coconut oil (or cacao butter, melted)

1/2 teaspoon baking soda

1/2 teaspoon baking powder

2 teaspoons ground ginger

1 teaspoon ground cinnamon

1 teaspoon vanilla

1/2 teaspoon ground cloves

1/2 teaspoon ground black pepper

1/4 teaspoon Celtic sea salt

Natural sarsaparilla or root beer beverage, or nut milk (optional)

INSTRUCTIONS

1. Preheat oven to 350 degrees F. Line sheet pan with parchment or baking mat.

2. Add dates, honey or agave and eggs to food processor or high-speed blender. Process until thick smooth mixture forms, about 2 minutes.

3. Add almond flour, oil or butter, baking soda and powder, salt and spices to processor. Process until thick mixture comes together, about 1 minute. Add sarsaparilla, root beer or nut milk to thin as necessary. Batter should resemble thick cookie dough.

4. From rounds and place on prepares sheet pan. Flatten into disks.

5. Bake 10 - 15 minutes, until browned around edges and cooked through, but still soft.

6. Remove from oven and let cool at about 10 minutes.

7. Transfer to serving dish and serve warm. Or cool completely and serve room temperature.

Basic Banana Bread

Prep Time: 5 minutes

Cook Time: 40 minutes

Servings: 8

INGREDIENTS

1 cup almond flour

1/4 cup coconut flour

2 overripe bananas

2 cage-free eggs

1/4 cup raw honey (or agave, date butter or stevia)

1/4 cup coconut oil (or coconut or cacao butter, melted) (or unsweetened applesauce or nut butter)

1 tablespoon baking powder

2 teaspoons ground cinnamon

1/2 teaspoon ground nutmeg

1 teaspoon vanilla

1/2 teaspoon Celtic sea salt

INSTRUCTIONS

1. Preheat oven to 350 degrees F. Coat small or medium loaf pan with coconut oil.
2. Peel bananas and add to medium mixing bowl. Beat with hand mixer or whisk. Add eggs, oil or butter, and sweetener. Beat well, about 1 - 2 minutes.

3. In separate bowl, blend flours, baking powder, salt and spices. Pour banana mixture into flour mixture and stir to combine.

4. Pour batter into prepared loaf pan and bake for 30 - 40 minutes, or until browned and firm in the center.

5. Remove from oven and set aside to cool.

6. Slice and serve warm. Or allow to cool completely and serve room temperature.

Scrumptious Cinnamon Buns

Prep Time: 15 minutes

Cook Time: 30 minutes

Servings: 8

INGREDIENTS

Rolls

3 cups almond flour

3 cage-free eggs

1/2 cup date butter (or raw honey or agave)

1/4 cup ground chia seed (or flax meal)

1/4 cup tapioca flour (or arrowroot powder)

1/4 cup nut milk

2 teaspoons baking powder

1/4 teaspoon Celtic sea salt

Coconut oil (for cooking)

Filling

1/4 cup ghee (or cacao or coconut butter, melted)

3/4 cup dried pitted dates

2 tablespoons ground cinnamon

Icing

1/2 cup raw honey (or date butter or agave)

1/2 cup full-fat coconut milk

INSTRUCTIONS

1. Preheat oven to 350 degrees F. Line cake pan or round baking dish with coconut oil. Cover cutting board with parchment and coat heavily with coconut oil.

2. For *Rolls*, heat nut milk in small pan over medium heat. Whisk in tapioca until combined. Remove from heat.

3. Add eggs to food processor or high-speed blender. Process until pale and silky, about 2 minutes. Add sweetener, chia meal, baking powder and salt. Process until combined, about 1 minute.

4. Add egg mixture and tapioca mixture to medium mixing bowl. Beat in almond flour 1 cup at a time with hand mixer or whisk.

5. Place dough on prepared parchment. Oil hands to prevent sticking and press dough into large 1/2 inch thick rectangle.

6. For *Filling*, add ghee or butter, dates and cinnamon to clean food processor or high-speed blender. Process until finely ground or smooth, about 1 - 2 minutes.

7. Sprinkle *Filling* over dough. Roll dough into log along short edge using parchment paper. Use sharp knife or floss to slice log into rolls.

8. Place *Rolls* in prepared cake pan or baking dish. Bake about 15 minutes.

9. For *Icing*, add sweetener and coconut milk to clean food processor or high-speed blender. Process until well combined, about 1 minute.

10. Remove *Rolls* from oven and carefully pour Icing over *Rolls*. Place back in oven and bake 10 - 15 minutes, until *Rolls* are cooked through and *Icing* is warm.

11. Remove from oven and serve hot. Or let cool about 5 minutes and serve room warm.

Yummy Strawberry Rhubarb Pie

Prep Time: 10 minutes

Cook Time: 50 minutes

Servings: 12

INGREDIENTS

Crust

2 cups almond flour

1 cage-free egg

2 tablespoons coconut oil (or cacao butter or ghee)

1/4 teaspoon Celtic sea salt

Filling

1/4 cup tapioca flour (or arrowroot powder)

2 1/2 cups diced rhubarb (fresh or frozen)

2 1/2 cups fresh strawberries (sliced)

3/4 cup raw honey (or agave or date butter)

1/2 lemon

1 teaspoon ground cinnamon

1 teaspoon vanilla

INSTRUCTIONS

1. Preheat oven to 350 degrees F.
2. For *Crust*, blend almond flour and salt in small mixing bowl. Add egg and oil or butter. Mix until dough forms. Press into pie pan with hand or wooden spoon.

3. Bake *Crust* about 10 minutes.

4. For *Filling*, add strawberries and rhubarb to medium pot. Heat over medium-high heat and stir lightly. Zest *then* juice lemon into pot. Cook about 5 minutes to release juices.

5. Sift tapioca over fruit and stir to combine. Cook about 5 minutes, then add sweetener, vanilla and cinnamon. Remove from heat.

6. Remove *Crust* from oven and carefully pour in *Filling*.

7. Bake about 35 - 40 minutes, or until fruit is set.

8. Remove from oven and let cool about 20 minutes.

9. Slice and serve warm. Or let cool completely and serve room temperature.

Sweet Raisin Pecan Cake

Prep Time: 10 minutes

Cook Time: 40 minutes

Servings: 12

INGREDIENTS

6 cage-free eggs

1 cup coconut flour

1/2 cup date butter (or agave or raw honey)

1/2 cup unsweetened applesauce

1/2 cup nut milk

1/4 cup coconut oil (or cacao or coconut butter, melted)

1 cup pecans

1/2 cup raisins

1 teaspoon vanilla

1 teaspoon baking soda

1 teaspoon baking powder

1/2 teaspoon Celtic sea salt

INSTRUCTIONS
1. Preheat oven to 350 degrees F. Coat Bundt pan with coconut oil.
2. Add egg whites to food processor or high-speed blender. Process until light and frothy, about 1 - 2 minutes.
3. Add egg yolks, coconut flour, sweetener, applesauce, nut milk, oil or butter, baking soda and powder, vanilla and salt. Process until

well combined batter comes together, about 2 minutes. Chop pecans and stir in with raisins.

4. Pour batter into prepared Bundt pan and bake for about 40 minutes, until golden brown and toothpick inserted halfway between edge and center of pan comes out clean.

5. Remove from oven and allow to cool at least 10 minutes.

6. Place serving dish over pan, invert and release cake to plate.

7. Slice and serve warm. Or let cool completely and serve room temperature.

Slim Cranberry Almond Cookies

Time: 10 minutes

Cook Time: 15 minutes

Servings: 12

INGREDIENTS

1 1/2 cups almond flour

1 cage-free egg

1/4 cup coconut oil (or cacao or coconut butter)

1/4 cup raw honey (or agave or date butter)

1/4 cup almond butter

1/4 cup almonds

1/4 cup dried cranberries

1/2 teaspoon baking powder

1 teaspoon vanilla

1/4 teaspoon Celtic sea salt

INSTRUCTIONS

1. Preheat oven to 350 degrees F. Line sheet pan with parchment or baking mat.
2. Sift flour, baking powder and salt into medium mixing bowl. Beat with whisk or hand mixer to lighten. Add egg, oil or butter, sweetener, almond butter, vanilla and salt. Mix well to form dough.
3. Chop almonds and add to bowl with cranberries. Mix to combine.

4. Shape dough into 12 balls and place on prepared baking sheet. Flatten slightly with hand or spatula.

5. Place in oven and bake 10 - 15 minutes, until golden brown along edges.

6. Remove from oven and let cool 5 minutes.

7. Serve warm. Or transfer to wire rack to cool completely and serve room temperature.

Pineapple Coconut Cake

Prep Time: 10 minutes

Cook Time: 45 minutes

Servings: 12

INGREDIENTS

6 cage-free eggs

3/4 cup coconut flour

1 cup flaked coconut

1 1/2 cups pineapple (diced)

1/2 cup raw honey (or agave or date butter)

1/2 cup coconut oil (or cacao or coconut butter, melted)

1 teaspoon baking soda

1 teaspoon baking powder

1 teaspoon vanilla

1/2 teaspoon Celtic sea salt

INSTRUCTIONS

1. Preheat oven to 350 degrees F. Lightly coat square or rectangular baking dish with coconut oil.
2. Add eggs to food processor or high-speed blender. Process until pale and lightened, about 2 minutes.
3. Add flour, coconut, pineapple, sweetener, oil or butter, baking soda, baking powder, vanilla and salt. Process until well combined, about 1 - 2 minutes.

4. Pour batter into prepared baking dish and bake about 45 minutes, until golden brown and firm in the center.

5. Remove from oven and allow to cool about 10 minutes.

6. Slice and serve warm. Or let cool completely and serve room temperature.

Mocha Brownie Bites

Prep Time: 5 minutes

Cook Time: 25 minutes

Servings: 16

INGREDIENTS

4 cage-free eggs

1 cup cocoa powder

1/4 cup coconut oil

1/4 cup full-fat coconut milk

1/4 cup sweetener*

2 teaspoons instant espresso (or instant coffee)

1 teaspoon vanilla

INSTRUCTIONS

1. Preheat oven to 350 degrees F. Lightly oil square baking dish or line with parchment.
2. Add eggs, coconut oil, coconut milk and sweetener to medium mixing bowl and beat with hand mixer or whisk. Sift in cocoa powder, espresso and vanilla. Beat until well combined.
3. Pour batter into prepared baking pan and bake for 20 - 25 minutes, until set.
4. Allow to cool completely.
5. Slice and serve room temperature. Or refrigerate and serve chilled.

* raw honey, agave nectar or maple syrup

Cinnamon Raisin Bread

Prep Time: 5 minutes

Cook Time: 20 minutes

Servings: 12

INGREDIENTS

3/4 cup coconut flour

3/4 cup almond flour

1/4 cup ground chia seed (or flax meal)

2 cage-free eggs

1/2 cup raisins

1/2 cup coconut oil

1/2 cup unsweetened applesauce

1/4 cup sweetener*

2 tablespoons ground cinnamon

1 teaspoon baking powder

1 teaspoon sea salt

1/2 teaspoon ground black pepper (optional)

INSTRUCTIONS

1. Preheat oven to 350 degrees F. Line baking pan with parchment or coat with coconut oil.

2. In large bowl, whisk eggs with hand mixer or whisk until frothy and light. Add coconut oil, sweetener and applesauce. Blend until combined.

3. Sift coconut and almond flour, chia meal, baking powder, salt and spices into wet ingredients. Beat until smooth and well combined. Stir in raisins.

4. Pour batter into prepared baking pan.

5. Bake for 20 - 25 minutes, or until golden brown and firm to the touch.

6. Remove from oven and let cool about 5 minutes.

7. Slice and serve warm. Or allow to cool completely and serve room temperature.

NOTE: Bake in oiled loaf pan for 40 - 45 minutes for **Cinnamon Raisin Bread** loaf.

stevia, raw honey or agave nectar

Easy Poppy Seed Muffins

Prep Time: 5 minutes

Cook Time: 20 minutes

Servings: 12

INGREDIENTS

6 eggs

1/2 cup coconut flour

1/4 cup coconut oil

1/4 cup sweetener*

1 teaspoon vanilla

1 teaspoon poppy seeds

1/2 teaspoon baking soda

Juice of 2 lemons

Zest of 2 lemons

INSTRUCTIONS

1. Preheat oven to 350 degrees F. Oil muffin pan or line with paper liners.
2. Zest, *then* juice 2 lemons. Add to large mixing bowl with eggs, coconut oil, sweetener and vanilla. Beat with hand mixer or whisk until well combined.
3. Sift coconut flour and baking soda into wet ingredients, and mix until smooth. Stir in poppy seeds.
4. Use ice cream scoop or tablespoon to pour batter into prepared muffin pan.

5. Place in oven and bake for about 20 minutes, or until golden around edges and toothpick inserted into middle comes out clean.
6. Remove from oven and let cool for 5 minutes.
7. Serve warm. Or allow to cool completely and serve room temperature.

raw honey or agave nectar

Blackberry Dumplings

Prep Time: 15 minutes

Cook Time: 20 minutes

Servings: 8

INGREDIENTS

Blackberry Filling

2 1/2 cups blackberries (fresh or frozen)

2 - 4 tablespoons sweetener*

2 tablespoons tapioca flour

1/2 teaspoon ground black pepper

Zest of 1/2 lemon

Dumplings

1/4 cup coconut flour

3/4 cup almond flour

3 tablespoons cold coconut oil

1 teaspoon baking powder

1/2 teaspoon ground cinnamon

1/4 teaspoon sea salt

2 cage-free eggs

2 tablespoon sweetener

1 teaspoon vanilla

Zest of 1/2 lemon

INSTRUCTIONS

1. For *Dumplings*, sift coconut flour, almond flour, baking powder and salt into small mixing bowl. Cut in cold coconut oil with fork until crumbly. Place in freezer for 10 minutes.

2. Preheat oven to 400 degrees F.

3. For *Blackberry Filling*, add blackberries, sweetener, black pepper and lemon zest to medium pot. Heat over medium heat and bring to simmer. Whisk in tapioca flour and simmer about 10 minutes.

4. Pour hot blackberries into casserole dish and place in hot oven.

5. In medium bowl, beat eggs, sweetener, lemon zest, cinnamon and vanilla. Add chilled flour mixture to eggs and mix until dough comes together.

6. Carefully remove dish from oven and drop 8 dumplings onto bubbling berries.

7. Return dish to oven and bake 15 - 20 min, until dumplings are golden, set and cooked through.

8. Remove dish from oven and allow to cool about 5 minutes.

9. Serve warm. Or allow to cool completely and serve room temperature.

*stevia, raw honey or agave nectar

Skinny Coconut Baked Donut

Prep Time: 5 minutes

Cook Time: 20 minutes

Servings: 6

INGREDIENTS

Donuts

1 3/4 cups almond flour

1 tablespoon coconut flour

2 eggs

1/3 cup coconut oil

1/4 cup unsweetened applesauce

1/4 cup sweetener*

2 tablespoons nut milk

2 teaspoons vanilla

3/4 teaspoon baking soda

1/2 teaspoon sea salt

Topping

1/2 cup flaked or shredded coconut

1/4 cup full-fat coconut milk

2 tablespoon sweetener

1/4 teaspoon vanilla

INSTRUCTIONS

1. Preheat oven to 350 degreesF. Lightly coat donut pan with coconut oil.

2. Add almond and coconut flours, baking soda and salt to food processor or high-speed blender. Process for 1 minute.

3. Add eggs, sweetener, coconut oil, applesauce, nut milk and vanilla. Process until light, thick batter forms, about 1 - 2 minutes.

4. Pour batter into donut pan until wells are 3/4 full.

5. Place in oven and bake for about 20 minutes, until dough is set and lightly browned.

6. For *Topping*, combine coconut milk, sweetener and vanilla in small mixing bowl.

7. Remove pan from oven at let cool about 5 minutes. Then remove donuts from pan.

8. Dip donuts in coconut icing then sprinkle with flaked or shredded coconut.

9. Transfer decorated donuts to serving dish.

10. Serve warm. Or let cool completely and serve room temperature.

NOTE: Bake in 8 mini cake pans or specialty cake pop pans lightly coated with coconut oil for fillable donuts or donut holes if you do not have a donut pan.

* stevia, raw honey or agave nectar

Delicious Apple Pastries

Prep Time: 20 minutes

Cook Time: 20 minutes

Servings: 4

INGREDIENTS

Crust

2 cups almond flour

2 cage-free eggs

3 tablespoons coconut oil

1 tablespoon sweetener*

1/2 teaspoon baking soda

1/2 teaspoon baking powder

1 teaspoon ground cinnamon

1/4 teaspoon sea salt

Filling

2 sweet apples

1/4 cup water

1 teaspoon tapioca flour

1 tablespoon ground cinnamon

1/2 teaspoon ground nutmeg

1 teaspoon vanilla

2 tablespoons sweetener * (optional)

2 tablespoons raisins (optional)

2 tablespoons chopped walnuts (optional)

DIRECTIONS

1. For *Crust*, sift almond flour into medium mixing bowl. Add baking soda and powder, cinnamon and salt.

2. Whisk eggs and sweetener in small mixing bowl, then add to flour mixture and combine. Slowly add coconut oil until malleable dough comes together.

3. Roll in plastic wrap or wrap tightly in parchment and refrigerate for 15 minutes.

4. Preheat oven to 400 degrees. Line sheet pan with parchment or baking mat. Cover cutting board with parchment. Heat medium pan over medium-high heat.

5. For *Filling*, peel and dice apples. Add apples to hot pan with water, tapioca, cinnamon, nutmeg, and sweetener and spices (optional).

6. Stir and simmer for about 5 - 8 minutes, until apples are tender and thick glaze forms. Remove from heat and add raisins and chopped walnuts (optional).

7. Remove dough from refrigerator. Roll dough out on parchment covered cutting board to about 1/8 inch thick square with rolling pin. Use sharp knife or pizza cutter to cut dough into 4 squares.

8. Scoop equal portions of *Filling* into center of one side of each dough square. Fold bare half of dough over filled half. Press edges together and secure seal, letting any trapped air escape. Repeat with remaining dough.

9. Arrange pies on lined sheet pan and bake 15 - 20 minutes, or until dough is golden and cooked through.

10. Serve immediately. Or allow to cool and serve room temperature.

stevia, raw honey or agave nectar

Healthy Lemon Coconut Bars

Prep Time: 15 minutes

Cook Time: 30 minutes

Servings: 12

INGREDIENTS

Crust

1/2 cup raw cashews

2/3 cup coconut flour

2 cage-free eggs

2 tablespoons coconut oil

2 tablespoons sweetener*

1 tablespoon flaked coconut

1 teaspoon fresh lemon juice

1/2 teaspoon baking soda

1/2 teaspoon vanilla

Filling

2 cage-free eggs

2 cage-free egg yolks

1 cup fresh lemon juice (about 6 lemons)

1/2 cup sweetener*

1/3 - 1/2 cup flaked coconut

2 tablespoons coconut flour

1 teaspoon lemon zest

INSTRUCTIONS

1. Preheat oven to 350 degrees F. Lightly coat rectangular baking dish with coconut oil, or line with parchment.

2. For *Crust*, add cashews and coconut to food processor or bullet blender and process until finely ground. Add remaining *Crust* ingredients to food processor and pulse until dough comes together.

3. Press dough into bottom of baking dish, and slightly up the sides. Dock crust with fork to prevent bubbling.

4. Place crust in oven and bake for 8 - 10 minutes.

5. For *Filling*, beat eggs, egg yolks, lemon juice, lemon zest and sweetener with hand mixer or whisk in medium bowl.

6. Sift in coconut flour and beat to combine. Let mixture sit for 5 minutes. Add flaked coconut and beat again to combine.

7. Pour *Filling* over par baked crust. Place in oven and bake 20 minutes, until center is set but still slightly jiggly.

8. Remove from oven and let cool for 20 minutes. Refrigerate about 20 minutes, until fully set and chilled.

9. Serve chilled or room temperature.

* raw honey or agave nectar

Cocoa Spice Pinwheel Cookies

Prep Time: 10 minutes

Cook Time: 20 minutes

Servings: 12

INGREDIENTS

2 cups almond flour

2 tablespoon sweetener*

1 egg

1 teaspoon vanilla

1/2 teaspoon baking powder

1/4 teaspoon sea salt

Filling

2 tablespoons cocoa powder

2 tablespoons sweetener*

2 teaspoons ground cinnamon

1 teaspoon ground black pepper

1/2 teaspoon vanilla

INSTRUCTIONS

1. Preheat oven to 300 degrees F. Line sheet pan with parchment or baking mat. Prepare 2 additional sheets of parchment.
2. Add flour, egg, sweetener, vanilla, baking powder and salt to medium bowl. Blend with wooden spoon, then knead with hand to form thick dough.

3. Divide dough in half. Place half of dough in small mixing bowl. Add all *Filling* ingredients to bowl and mix until well combined.

4. Roll out each half of dough separately on parchment sheets. Roll into equal rectangles.

5. Place *Filling* rectangle on top of plain dough. Use parchment to help roll dough tightly along long edge into log.

6. Use sharp knife to cut log into 1/4 round slices. Place cookies on prepared sheet pan and bake about 10 minutes, until edges are golden brown.

7. Remove from oven and let cool about 5 minutes.

8. Serve warm. Or let cool completely and serve room temperature.

*raw honey, agave nectar or maple syrup

Chocolate Pecan Shortbread Cookies

Prep Time: 5 minutes

Cook Time: 20 minutes

Servings: 12

INGREDIENTS

1 1/2 cups almond flour

1 1/2 cup pecans

1/4 cup cocoa powder

1/4 cup coconut oil (or melted cacao butter)

1/4 cup sweetener*

1 teaspoons vanilla

1/4 teaspoon baking soda

1/2 teaspoon sea salt

INSTRUCTIONS

1. Preheat oven to 300 degrees F. Line sheet pan with parchment or baking mat.
2. Add 1 cup pecans to food processor or high-speed blender and process until finely ground.
3. Add ground pecans to medium mixing bowl. Sift in almond flour, cocoa, baking soda and salt.
4. Chop remaining pecans and add to small mixing bowl. Add coconut oil or melted cacao butter, sweetener and vanilla to pecans. Mix to combine.
5. Pour wet mixture into dry ingredients and mix to form dough.

6. Use mini ice cream scoop or tablespoon to drop portions of dough onto prepared sheet pan.
7. Place in oven and bake 20 minutes, or until lightly browned.
8. Remove from oven and let cool at least 5 minutes.
9. Let cool completely and serve room temperature. Or serve warm.

*raw honey, agave nectar or maple syrup

Red Velvet Bars

Prep Time: 20 minutes

Cook Time: 25 minutes

Servings: 16

INGREDIENTS

4 eggs

1/2 cup cocoa powder

1/2 cup almond flour

1/4 cup coconut oil

1/4 cup full-fat coconut milk

1/4 cup sweetener*

Juice of 1 beet

1 teaspoon vanilla

Topping

Coconut cream (settled from 1 can full-fat coconut milk)

2 - 4 tablespoons sweetener*

1/2 teaspoon vanilla

INSTRUCTIONS

1. Preheat oven to 350 degrees F. Lightly oil square baking dish or line with parchment.

2. Juice beet and add to medium mixing bowl. Add cocoa powder, eggs, coconut oil, coconut milk, sweetener and vanilla. Beat with hand mixer or whisk until well combined.

3. Pour batter into prepared baking pan and bake for 25 minutes, until set.

4. For *Topping*, beat coconut cream in medium mixing bowl until slightly thickened. Add sweetener and vanilla. Continue to beat until full thickened and fluffy, about 5 minutes.

5. Remove dish from oven and allow to cool. Frost with *Topping*.

6. Slice and serve room temperature. Or refrigerate and serve chilled.

* raw honey, agave nectar or maple syrup

Wild Mince Meat Pie

Prep Time: 20 minutes

Cook Time: 30 minutes

Servings: 8

INGREDIENTS

Crust

4 cups almond flour

2 eggs

1/4 cup coconut oil

1/2 teaspoon sea salt

Filling

12 oz grass-fed beef

2 sweet apples

2 tart apples

1 cup beef stock

1/4 cup sweetener*

Juice of 1 orange

Zest of 1 orange

1/4 cup arrowroot powder

1/4 cup apple cider vinegar

1 cup raisins

1/2 cup dried pitted dates

1/2 cup dried pitted prunes

1/2 cup dried cherries

2 teaspoons ground cinnamon

1 teaspoon ground nutmeg

1/2 teaspoon ground cloves

1/2 teaspoon ground black pepper

1/2 teaspoon salt

INSTRUCTIONS

1. Preheat oven to 350 degrees F. Heat large pot over medium-high heat and lightly coat with coconut oil. Lightly oil pie plate. Prepare 4 sheets of parchment.

2. Place beef in hot oiled pan and brown on each side for about 5 - 7 minutes, until just cooked through. Remove beef and set aside. Add beef stock to pot.

3. Mix all *Crust* ingredients together in medium bowl until dough forms. Divide dough in half and use rolling pin to roll dough between two parchment sheets into circles to fit about 1 inch over pie plate.

4. Press one dough circle into pie plate. Crimp edges to create small lip. Bake for 5 minutes, then remove and set aside.

5. Peel, core and grate or dice apples. Add to beef stock with sweetener, zest and juice of orange, vinegar, raisins, cherries, spices and salt. Dice beef, prunes and dates, and add to pot. Stir in arrowroot powder and thicken for a few minutes.

6. Once mixture comes together pour into par baked pie shell. Top with second dough sheet and crimp edges to fit into bottom crust.

7. Use sharp knife to slice top crust a few times for venting.

8. Bake pie for 30 minutes, or until crust is golden brown.

9. Remove from oven and allow to cool for about 20 minutes.

10. Slice and serve warm. Or allow to cool completely and serve room temperature.

stevia, raw honey or agave nectar

Baked Peaches

Prep Time: 5 minutes

Cook Time: 25 minutes

Servings: 4

INGREDIENTS

2 ripe peaches

1/4 cup walnuts

1/4 cup dried cranberries

2 tablespoons sweetener*

Juice of 1 orange

Zest of 1 orange

1 teaspoon cinnamon

1/2 teaspoon nutmeg

1/2 teaspoon ground allspice

INSTRUCTIONS

1. Preheat oven to 375 degrees F.
2. Slice peaches in half and remove pit. Place peach halves into glass or ceramic baking dish just big enough for them to fit snuggly.
3. Chop walnuts and toss with cranberries, sweetener, spices, juice and zest of orange in small bowl.
4. Fill peach halves with fruit and nut mixture. Pour excess liquid over peaches.
5. Bake in oven for about 20 - 25 minutes, until peaches are soften and lightly browned.

6. Remove from oven and let cool about 5 minutes.

7. Serve warm or room temperature.

stevia, raw honey or agave nectar

Tiramisu

Prep Time: 20 minutes*

Cook Time: 10 minutes

Servings: 8

INGREDIENTS

Lady Fingers

1/3 cup coconut flour

3 tablespoons arrowroot powder

4 eggs

1/4 cup sweetener**

1/2 teaspoon baking powder

1/2 teaspoon vanilla

2 tablespoons instant espresso (or instant coffee)

3/4 cup water

2 tablespoons cocoa powder

Cashew Mascarpone

2 cups cashews

2 tablespoons sweetener**

1 teaspoon lemon juice

1 teaspoon vanilla

Water

INSTRUCTIONS

1. *Soak 2 cups cashews in water overnight. Drain and rinse.

2. Preheat oven to 400 degrees F. Line two sheet pans with parchment paper. Fit pastry bag with 1/2 inch round tube, or cut 1/4 inch corner off sturdy kitchen storage bag (like Ziploc®).

3. Beat egg yolks, 1/4 cup sweetener and 1/2 teaspoon vanilla until thick and pale.

4. In separate bowl beat egg whites to stiff peaks with hand mixer or whisk in medium bowl. Fold half of egg whites into egg yolk mixture. Then sift in coconut flour, arrowroot powder and baking powder. Fold in remaining egg whites.

5. Scoop batter into pastry bag or storage bag. Place in tall wide contain and fold open end of bag over edge of container for greater ease.

6. Pipe 5 inch lady fingers onto parchment lined sheet pans about 2 inches apart. Bake for 8 minutes.

7. Remove cookies from oven and transfer full parchment sheet onto wire rack to cool completely. Do not try to remove warm cookies from parchment.

8. Process soaked cashews in food processor or bullet blender with sweetener, lemon juice, vanilla, and just enough water to smooth.

9. Bring 3/4 cup water just under a boil. Dissolve instant espresso or coffee in water and add to shallow dish.

10. Remove cooled lady fingers form parchment. Dip and roll each cookie in espresso, then arrange in single layer in glass baking dish. Cut cookies to fit into tight layer.

11. Dollop and spread on half of *Cashew Mascarpone*. Then add another layer of espresso dipped lady fingers. Top with last half of *Cashew Mascarpone* and sift on cocoa powder.
12. *Refrigerate at least 30 - 60 minutes.
13. Slice and serve chilled.

*stevia, raw honey or agave nectar

Chocolate Almond Biscotti

Prep Time: 15 minutes

Cook Time: 35* minutes

Servings: 6

INGREDIENTS

1 cup almond flour

1/2 cup coconut flour

1/2 cup sweetener*

1/3 cup almonds

2 tablespoons cocoa powder

1 teaspoon vanilla

1/2 teaspoon baking soda

1/4 teaspoon sea salt

INSTRUCTIONS

1. Preheat oven to 350 degrees F. Line sheet pan with parchment paper. Heat medium pan over medium heat.

2. Add almonds to hot dry pan and toast for about 5 minutes, until aromatic. Stir frequently. Remove from heat and set aside.

3. In medium mixing bowl, blend almond flour, coconut flour, cocoa powder, baking soda and salt with hand mixer or whisk.

4. Beat in sweetener and vanilla until well combined and thick, sticky dough forms. Mix in toasted almonds with wooden spoon.

5. Form dough into flattened, uniform mound about 1 inch thick on sheet pan. Pat down mound to keep any almonds from sticking out.

6. Bake for about 15 minutes . Remove and allow to cool for about 15 minutes.

7. Use a very sharp serrated knife to carefully cut biscotti log into 1/2 - 2/3 inch slices. Hold onto the mound and cut on a diagonal. If it becomes crumbly, stick it back together.

8. Lace slice on sides and return to oven for 15 minutes.

9. Try to cut so that you're holding on to the edges of the log to keep it from crumbling. If parts come apart, you can stick them back together as the mixture is still kind of sticky.

10. Lay the biscotti flat and return to oven for 15 minutes.

11. *Turn oven off and leave oven door open a crack. Allow the biscotti to cool and dry for at least 2 hours.

12. Serve room temperature.

*raw honey, agave nectar, maple syrup, or any combination

Ginger Mango Sherbet

Prep Time: 5* minutes

Cook Time: 15 minutes

Servings: 4

INGREDIENTS

1 cup almond milk

1 cup coconut milk

2 ripe mangos

2 oz fresh ginger juice (about 8 inch bunch ginger root)

Juice of lime half

Zest of lime half

1 teaspoon vanilla

Bunch fresh mint

INSTRUCTIONS

1. *Freeze ice cream maker canister overnight before to make sure it is cold enough.

2. Add whole peeled ginger root to food processor. Or juice ginger and add to medium mixing bowl. Add mint leaves.

3. Slice, pit and peel mangos. Add to food processor or bullet blender with almond milk. Blend or process until smooth, then strain into medium mixing bowl.

4. Add coconut milk, juice and zest of half a lime, and vanilla. Mix well with whisk or hand mixer.

5. Turn on ice cream maker first, then carefully pour in mango mixture as ice cream maker paddle rotates.

6. Freeze for about 15 - 20 minutes. Then transfer frozen custard to serving dishes.

7. Serve immediately.

Pineapple Upside Down Cake

Prep Time: 15 minutes

Cook Time: 30 minutes

Servings: 12

INGREDIENTS

2 cups almond flour

8 - 12 slices organic canned pineapple in juice

8 - 12 pitted cherries

1/4 cup sweetener*

3 eggs

1/4 cup coconut oil

1/2 cup organic pineapple juice (reserved from can)

2 teaspoons baking soda

2 teaspoons vanilla

1/2 teaspoon sea salt

INSTRUCTIONS
1. Preheat oven to 350 degrees F. Line 9x13 baking dish with parchment paper, or coat with coconut oil.
2. Arrange pineapple slices and cherries on bottom of baking dish. Place in oven while you prepare the batter.
3. Beat egg whites to stiff peaks with hand mixer or whisk in medium mixing bowl. About 7 - 10 minutes.
4. In large mixing bowl, mix yolks, olive oil, sweetener, pineapple juice and vanilla.

5. Sift almond flour, baking soda and salt into yolk mixture. Beat until well combined.

6. Fold egg whites into batter until evenly combined.

7. Remove hot baking pan from oven, and spread light batter over pineapple and cherries. Smooth top with spatula.

8. Bake for 25 - 30 minutes, or until cake golden brown and firm but springy in the center. A toothpick inserted into the center should come out clean.

9. Remove pan from oven and allow to cool for 15 minutes. Turn cake out onto serving dish and remove parchment. Or scrape any stuck fruit from the pan and place back on cake.

10. Allow to cool another 15 minutes before serving. Serve room temperature or warm.

NOTE: For **Pineapple Upside Dow Cupcakes** , add a pineapple slice and cherry to muffin pan lined with paper liners or coated with coconut oil, then fill cups 2/3 full with batter and bake about 20 minutes.

stevia, raw honey or agave nectar

Cashew Chocolate Mousse

Prep Time: 5 minutes*

Servings: 2

INGREDIENTS

2 cups raw cashews

1/2 unsweetened flaked or shredded coconut

1/2 cup dried pitted dates

1/4 cup raw cacao powder

1 teaspoon vanilla

3 cups water

INSTRUCTIONS

1. *Soaked cashews and dates in 2 cups of water overnight. Separately soak coconut in 1 cup water overnight.

2. Add soaked coconut and water to high-speed blender. Process on high until smooth, about 1 minute.

3. Strain coconut mixture through nut milk bag or a few layers of cheese cloth. Squeeze out all excess liquid. Reserve coconut milk and set aside. Dry excess coconut, process until finely ground, and use as coconut flour.

4. Add drained soaked cashews and dates to clean food processor or high-speed blender with cacao powder and vanilla. Add 1/4 cup coconut milk and process on high until smooth and creamy. Add more coconut milk as necessary to reach desired consistency.

5. Pour mousse into serving dishes and serve immediately. Or freeze 15 minutes to thicken.
6. Serve room temperature or chilled.

Sweet Cinnamon Pretzel

Prep Time: 10 minutes

Cook Time: 20 minutes

Servings: 4

INGREDIENTS

Cinnamon Pretzel

1 cup coconut flour

1/2 cup tapioca flour/starch

1/2 cup coconut oil

1/2 cup water

2 dried dates

1 egg

2 tablespoon apple cider vinegar

1/2 teaspoon baking soda

1/2 teaspoon baking powder

2 teaspoons ground cinnamon

1/2 teaspoon vanilla

1/2 teaspoon ground ginger

1/2 teaspoon sea salt

Coconut Sweet Cream

1/4 cup full-fat coconut milk

2 tablespoons sweetener

1 tablespoon lemon juice

1/2 teaspoon vanilla

INSTRUCTIONS

1. Preheat oven to 350 degrees F. Heat medium pot over medium-high heat. Line sheet pan with parchment or baking mat.

2. Add dates, coconut oil, water, vinegar and salt to food processor or bullet blender and process until smooth. Pour mixture into pot. Bring to a boil and remove from heat.

3. Whisk in tapioca flour. Stir with wooden spoon or soft spatula until mixture gels and comes together.

4. Stir in baking soda and baking powder. Continue mixing for a minute. Mixture will foam and expand. Let mixture sit and cool about 5 minutes.

5. Sift in coconut flour and spices. Mix partially, then beat in egg. Mix until combined. Excess coconut flour may sit in bottom of bowl.

6. Turn out dough onto cutting board dusted with any excess coconut flour from mixture. Knead dough for 2 minutes.

7. Cut dough into 4 equal portions. Roll out pieces into ropes and twist to form classic pretzel twist. Pinch together any crumbled dough.

8. Arrange pretzels on lined sheet pan. Brush with coconut oil or full-fat coconut milk.

9. Place sheet pan in oven and bake about 25 minutes, until cooked through.

10. For *Coconut Sweet Cream*, mix coconut milk, vanilla, sweetener and lemon juice with had mixer or whisk until thick and creamy. Transfer to serving dish.

11. Serve pretzels immediately with *Coconut Sweet Cream*. Or allow pretzels to cool and refrigerate sweet cream, and serve chilled.

*stevia, raw honey or agave nectar

Healthy Refrigerator Carrot Cake

Prep Time: 10 minutes*

Servings: 8

INGREDIENTS

Carrot Cake

2 - 3 large carrots

2 cups raw walnuts

1/2 cup raisins (or dried apricots)

1/2 cup flaked or shredded coconut

2 tablespoons raw pumpkin seeds

1/4 cup raw honey (or dried pitted dates)

1 teaspoon vanilla

1 teaspoon ground cinnamon

1/4teaspoon ground nutmeg

1/4 teaspoon ground ginger (optional)

Cashew Cream Icing

1 cup raw cashews

1/2 large lemon

2 tablespoons raw honey (or dried pitted dates)

1 teaspoon vanilla

Water

INSTRUCTIONS

1. *For *Cashew Cream Icing*, separately soak cashews and dates (if using) in enough water to cover for 2 hours. Drain dates. Drain and rinse cashews.

2. For *Carrot Cake*, add carrots to food processor or high-speed blender and pulse to roughly chop. Add all *Carrot Cake* ingredients and process until coarsely ground but still slightly chunky, about 1 minute.

3. Transfer mixture to cake or baking pan and press firmly with hands.

4. For *Cashew Cream Icing*, juice lemon and add to clean food processor or high-speed blender with soaked cashews, soaked dates or honey, and vanilla. Process until smooth, about 2 minutes. Add enough date soaking liquid or water to reach desired consistency.

5. Spread *Cashew Cream Icing* over *Carrot Cake* and place in refrigerator at least 2 hours.

6. Slice and serve chilled. Or allow to warm slightly and serve.

Ginger Punch Pudding

Prep Time: 20 minutes*

Servings: 2

INGREDIENTS

1 young coconut (about 1 cup coconut meat and 1 cup coconut water)

2 - 4 tablespoons raw honey (or pitted dates)

1 1/2 inch piece fresh ginger

1/2 teaspoon ground ginger

1 teaspoon vanilla

Water (optional)

INSTRUCTIONS

1. * Soak dates in enough water to cover for at least 4 hours, or overnight in refrigerator (if using). Drain.

2. Remove flesh from fresh coconut and add to high-speed blender with 1 cup coconut water. Process until well blended and fairly smooth, about 1 - 2 minutes.

3. Peel ginger and grate into processor. Add vanilla, ground ginger, and honey or dates. Process until smooth, about 1 minute.

4. Transfer to serving dish and serve immediately or refrigerate at least 20 minutes and serve chilled.

Quick Tropical Sorbet

Prep Time: 30 minutes

Servings: 4

INGREDIENTS

2 coconuts (or 1 cup flaked coconut)

3 ripe mangos

1 orange

INSTRUCTIONS

1. *Freeze ice cream maker canister overnight.
2. *Soak flaked coconut in 2 cups water overnight in refrigerator, if using.
3. Add soaked coconut and soaking liquid to high-speed blender. Process until well blended and fairly smooth, about 1 - 2 minutes.
4. Or remove flesh from fresh coconuts and add to high-speed blender with 2 cups water. Process until well blended and fairly smooth, about 1 - 2 minutes.
5. Strain mixture through nut milk bag, cheesecloth or strainer back into blender.
6. Reserve pulp and set aside to dry and dehydrate, then use as coconut flour.
7. Cut mangos in half and remove peel. Roughly chop and add to blender. Zest *then* juice orange. Add to processor and process until smooth, about 1 minute.

8. Turn on ice cream maker. Slowly pour mixture into running ice cream maker. Let machine run until ice cream forms, about 20 minutes.

9. Transfer to serving dish and serve immediately. Or store in airtight container in freezer.

Delicious Weeknight Dinners

Chicken Satay

Prep Time: 10 minutes*
Cook Time: 25 minutes
Servings: 4

INGREDIENTS

16 oz (1 lb) boneless skinless chicken

12 wooden skewers (soaked in water for 1 hour)

Marinade

1 tablespoon pure fish sauce (or liquid aminos or coconut Aminos)

2 inch piece fresh ginger rot

1 garlic clove

Satay Sauce

13 oz (1 can) full-fat coconut milk

1/2 cup crunchy almond butter

1 tablespoon raw honey or agave nectar

1 tablespoon pure fish sauce (or tamari or coconut aminos)

1 teaspoon apple cider vinegar (or liquid aminos or coconut vinegar)

4 shallots

2 garlic cloves

2 inch piece fresh ginger root

2 small red chili peppers

1 1/2 tablespoons lime juice

Coconut oil (for cooking)

INSTRUCTIONS

1. *Cut chicken into 1 inch strips. For *Marinade*, peel and mince garlic and ginger. Add to medium mixing bowl with fish sauce and whisk. Add chicken and toss with until coated. Cover and set aside to marinate for 1 hour.

2. *Soak wooden skewers in water in shallow dish for 1 hour.

3. Heat medium pan or wok over medium heat and add 1 tablespoon coconut oil.

4. For *Satay Sauce*, peel and mince shallots, garlic and ginger. Slice peppers. Add to hot pan and sauté until softened, about 5 - 8 minutes.

5. Reduce heat to low. Add almond butter, coconut milk, honey, fish sauce, vinegar and lime juice. Whisk until blended. Gently simmer for 10 minutes. Remove from heat, but keep warm.

6. Preheat outdoor grill or griddle pan over medium-high heat. Lightly coat with coconut oil.

7. Pierce marinated chicken strips with soaked skewers. Pour some *Satay Sauce* over chicken and brush lightly with marinade brush to coat. Transfer remaining *Satay Sauce* to serving dish.

8. Grill chicken on preheated grill until just cooked through, about 3 minutes per side. Turn over skewers halfway through cooking. Do not overcook.

9. Remove skewers from heat and transfer to serving dish. Serve with *Satay Sauce*.

Skinny Orange Chicken

Prep Time: 10 minutes

Cook Time: 10 minutes

Servings: 2

INGREDIENTS

12 oz (3/4 lb) boneless skinless chicken

1/2 cup almond flour

1 teaspoon flax meal

1 cage-free egg

1 green onion (scallion)

1/4 teaspoon cayenne pepper

1/2 teaspoon paprika

1/2 teaspoon ground black pepper

1/2 teaspoon Celtic sea salt

Coconut oil (for cooking)

Water

Orange Sauce

3 oranges (or tangerines or Clementines)

2 tablespoons raw honey (or agave)

1 tablespoon tamari (or liquid aminos or coconut aminos)

1 small garlic clove

1/2 inch piece fresh ginger

1/4 teaspoon ground black pepper

Water

INSTRUCTIONS

1. For *Orange Sauce*, zest 2 oranges, *then* juice all oranges into small pot. Peel and mince garlic and ginger. Add to pot with honey, tamari and pepper. Add 1/2 cup water.

2. Heat small pot over medium heat and bring to simmer. Simmer until *Orange Sauce* is reduced by half, about 5 minutes. Stir frequently. Remove from heat and set aside.

3. Heat medium pan over medium-high heat. Lightly coat pan with coconut oil.

4. In a shallow dish, blend almond meal, flax meal, salt and spices.

5. Whisk egg and 1 teaspoon water in separate shallow dish.

6. Cut chicken into 1 inch pieces. Dip chicken into egg wash, then dredge in seasoned almond meal.

7. Carefully place coated chicken pieces into hot oil and fry about 2 - 3 minutes, until golden brown and cooked through. Turn with tongs halfway through cooking.

8. Drain cooked chicken on paper towel, then transfer to medium mixing bowl. Pour *Orange Sauce* over chicken and toss to coat. Transfer to serving dish.

9. Slice scallions and sprinkle over dish. Serve hot.

Cashew Chicken

Prep Time: 5 minutes

Cook Time: 10 minutes

Servings: 2

INGREDIENTS

12 oz (3/4 lb) boneless skinless chicken

1/2 cup raw cashews

1/2 small onion (white or yellow)

1/2 red bell pepper

1/2 green bell pepper

1 small celery stalk

2 tablespoons tamari (or coconut aminos or apple cider vinegar)

1 teaspoon raw honey (or agave or date butter)

1 garlic clove

1/2 inch piece fresh ginger

1/4 teaspoon ground black pepper

1/2 teaspoon Celtic sea salt

Bacon fat or coconut oil (for cooking)

INSTRUCTIONS

1. Heat large pan or wok over medium heat. Lightly coat with bacon fat or coconut oil.

2. Peel and mince garlic and ginger. Remove seeds, stems and veins from peppers, then roughly chop. Dice carrot. Slice celery.

3. Roughly chop chicken and season with salt and pepper.

4. Add garlic and ginger to hot oiled pan or wok. Sauté about 1 minute, until fragrant. Add seasoned chicken add sauté until browned, about 2 minutes. Transfer chicken to small bowl and set aside.

5. Add veggies to hot oiled pan. Sauté until tender and lightly browned, about 2 minutes. Add tamari, honey and cashews. Sauté until veggies are just cooked, but still crisp.

6. Add chicken back to pan and heat until just cooked through, about 2 minutes.

7. Transfer to serving dish and serve hot.

Spicy Hunan Beef and Broccoli

Prep Time: 20 minutes

Cook Time: 10 minutes

Servings: 2

INGREDIENTS

12 oz (3/4 lb) beef sirloin

1/2 head broccoli

2 carrots

1 tablespoon tamari (or coconut aminos)

1 tablespoon dry sherry (or pure fish sauce or apple cider vinegar)

1 garlic clove

1/2 inch piece fresh ginger

1/2 teaspoon sesame seeds (optional)

Coconut oil (for cooking)

Sauce

1 tablespoon Asian chili paste

3 teaspoons tamari (or coconut aminos)

3 teaspoons chicken broth (or beef broth)

3 teaspoons dry sherry (or pure fish sauce or apple cider vinegar)

1 teaspoon raw honey (or agave)

1/2 teaspoon arrowroot flour

1/2 teaspoon sesame oil

2 garlic cloves

1/4 teaspoon fresh ground black pepper

INSTRUCTIONS

1. Cut beef against the grain into thin slices. Add to small mixing with tamari and sherry. And toss to coat. Set aside to marinate for 20 minutes.

2. For Sauce, peel and mince garlic. Add to small mixing bowl with chili paste, tamari, broth, sherry, honey, arrowroot, sesame oil and pepper. Mix to combine. Set aside.

3. Roughly chop broccoli into pieces. Slice carrots diagonally. Peel and mince garlic and ginger. Set aside.

4. Heat medium pan or wok over medium heat. Add 1 tablespoon coconut oil to hot pan.

5. Add marinated beef to hot pan in single layer. Let sear 1 minute on each side, undisturbed. Transfer to medium dish and set aside.

6. Add 1 tablespoon coconut oil to hot pan. Add garlic and ginger and sauté about 1 minute. Add broccoli and carrots. Sauté until lightly browned and softened, about 3 - 4 minutes. Stir frequently.

7. Add beef back to pan with *Sauce* and sesame seeds. Sauté until veggies are tender and beef is cooked through, about 2 minutes.

8. Transfer to serving dish and serve hot.

Meaty Texas Chili

Prep Time: 5 minutes

Cook Time: 40 minutes

Servings: 4

INGREDIENTS

16 oz (1 lb) lean grass-fed ground beef (or elk, bison, turkey or chicken)

15 oz (1 can) organic tomato sauce

29 oz (2 cans) organic diced tomatoes

1 cup water

1 cup cashews

1 small onion

1 bell pepper

2 cloves garlic

2 tablespoons chili powder

1 1/2 tablespoons smoked paprika (or paprika)

1 tablespoon ground cumin

1 teaspoon Mexican oregano (or dried oregano)

1 teaspoon ground black pepper

1/2 teaspoon cayenne pepper

1 teaspoon Celtic sea salt

1 tablespoon coconut oil

INSTRUCTIONS

1. Heat medium pot over medium-high heat. Add 1 tablespoon coconut oil to hot pan.

2. Peel onion and garlic. Remove stems, seeds and veins from bell pepper. Roughly chop and add to food processor or high-speed blender. Pulse until finely minced.

3. Add minced veggies to hot skillet and sauté for about 1 minute. Add ground beef and spices. Brown beef for about 5 minutes. Stir with whisk to break up meat well, or wooden spoon to keep beef chunkier.

4. Add whole cans of diced tomatoes and tomato sauce, and water. Stir to combine.

5. Bring to a simmer, then reduce heat to medium and cover pot loosely with lid to prevent splatter. Simmer about 30 minutes. Stir occasionally.

6. Remove from heat and transfer to serving dish. Use large serving spoon or ladle to serve hot.

Spicy Meatball Marinara

Prep Time: 5 minutes

Cook Time: 20 minutes

Servings: 4

INGREDIENTS

Meatballs

16 oz (1 lb) lean ground meat (beef, pork, chicken, turkey, bison, or any combination)

3/4 cup almond flour

1 cage-free egg

1/2 small onion (white, yellow or red)

1/2 teaspoon garlic powder

1/2 teaspoon cayenne pepper

1 teaspoon dried parsley

1 teaspoon dried oregano

1 teaspoon paprika

1 teaspoon red pepper flakes

1 teaspoon ground black pepper

1 teaspoon Celtic sea salt

1 tablespoon coconut oil

1 sprig fresh basil (for garnish, optional)

Tomato Sauce

14.5 oz (1 can) organic diced tomatoes

8 oz (1 can) organic tomato sauce

1 garlic clove

1/2 teaspoon dried oregano

1/2 teaspoon dried basil

1/2 teaspoon red pepper flakes

1/2 teaspoon ground black pepper

1 teaspoon coconut oil

INSTRUCTIONS

1. Heat large pan over medium heat. Add 1 tablespoon coconut oil to hot pan. Heat medium saucepan over medium heat. Add 1 teaspoon coconut oil.

2. For *Tomato Sauce*, peel garlic and mince. Add to medium saucepan and sauté until just golden, about 30 seconds. Add diced tomatoes, tomato sauce, salt and spices. Simmer about 5 - 10 minutes, stirring occasionally.

3. For *Meatballs*, peel onion process in food processor or high-speed blender, or finely grate.

4. Add to large mixing bowl. Add egg, ground meat, almond flour, spices and salt. Mix well with hands or large wooden spoon.

5. Form 24 meatballs with scoop or tablespoon, then roll in hands. Add meatballs to hot large pan and brown for 10 minutes. Turn with spatula or tongs to cook on all sides.

6. Add *Meatballs* to *Tomato Sauce* and simmer another 5 minutes.

7. Transfer *Meatballs* to serving dish. Top with simmering *Tomato Sauce*. Garnish with fresh basil (optional).

8. Serve hot.

Highland Sheppard's Pie

Prep Time: 20 minutes

Cook Time: 60 minutes

Servings: 4

INGREDIENTS

Meat Filling

24 oz (1 1/2 lbs) grass-fed ground lamb (or beef, bison, elk, etc.)

1 cup chicken broth or stock (or beef brother or stock, or red wine)

1 large onion (yellow or white)

2 carrots

6 - 10 asparagus stalks (about 1/2 cup chopped)

1/2 sweet potato (about 1/2 cup diced)

2 garlic cloves

1 tablespoon organic tomato paste

1 teaspoon tamari (or coconut aminos)

2 tablespoons tapioca flour (or arrow root powder)

1 sprig fresh rosemary

1 sprig fresh thyme

1/2 teaspoon ground black pepper (or ground white pepper)

1 teaspoon Celtic sea salt

Bacon fat or coconut oil (for cooking)

Parsnip Topping

4 medium parsnips

1/2 medium onion (yellow or white)

2 tablespoons cacao butter (or coconut oil)

2 cups water

3/4 teaspoon Celtic sea salt

1/2 ground white pepper (or ground black pepper) (optional)

INSTRUCTIONS

1. Heat medium pot over medium heat. Add 2 tablespoons bacon fat or coconut oil to hot pot.

2. For *Meat Filling*, peel and mince garlic. Peel and chop onion. Dice carrots and sweet potato. Chop asparagus. Add to hot oiled pot and sauté about 5 minutes.

3. Add lamb, salt and spices to veggies. Brown lamb and sauté another 5 minutes. Whisk in tapioca flour and cook another minute.

4. Remove rosemary and thymes leaves from stems and add to pot with stock, tomato paste and tamari. Let simmer and thicken about 12 minutes.

5. Preheat oven to 400 degrees F. Heat large pan with lid over medium heat. Add butter or oil to hot pan.

6. For *Parsnip Topping*, peel and mince or finely grate onion. Add to hot pan and sauté until translucent and aromatic, about 2 minutes.

7. Peel and slice or chop parsnips. Add to onions with water. Increase heat to high and bring to a simmer. Cover pan loosely with lid. Cook parsnips partially covered until softened and most of the water has evaporated, about 10 minutes.

8. Pour parsnips and onions into food processor or high-speed blender. Process until thick, smooth mixture forms. Add enough water to reach desired consistency. Set aside.

9. Transfer *Meat Filling* to baking or casserole dish. Top with *Parsnip Topping*. Smooth over or create design with offset spatula or back of spoon.

10. Bake about 25 minutes, until *Parsnip Topping* is golden.

11. Remove from oven and let cool at least 10 minutes. Serve warm.

Black Pepper Stew

Prep time: 15 minutes

Cook time: 3 hr 45 minutes

Serves: 6

INGREDIENTS

1 ½ lbs beef stew meat

1 onion

1 (14.5 oz) can no-salt added stewed tomatoes, undrained

¼ tsp Celtic sea salt

½ tsp ground black pepper

1 dried bay leaf

2 cups water

3 tbsp arrowroot powder

12 small sweet potatoes cut in half

30 baby-cut carrots

INSTRUCTIONS

1. Heat oven to 325 degrees. In a bowl, mix arrowroot in water and stir to a paste (if you're not using arrowroot, use 1 cup water instead). Cut the onion into 8 wedges and cut potatoes in half.
2. In ovenproof Dutch oven, mix beef, onion, tomatoes, Celtic sea salt, ground black pepper and bay leaf. Mix arrowroot-thickened water (or 1 cup water) into Dutch oven.
3. Cover and bake for 2 hours, stirring one time.

4. Stir in the potatoes and carrots. Cover and bake until beef and vegetables are tender, about 1 hr 45 min. Remove bay leaf and serve immediately, or chill 20 minutes and then serve.

Nuts & Turkey Burgers

Prep time: 10 minutes

Cook time: 6-12 minutes

Servings: 4

INGREDIENTS

16 oz ground turkey

1 cup walnuts

2 cloves garlic

1 onion

¼ tsp chipotle chili pepper powder

¼ tbsp smoked paprika

¼ tsp ground black pepper

INSTRUCTIONS

1. Chop walnuts into smaller pieces, about ⅛" cubes. Mince garlic and chop onion into small pieces, about ¼" pieces.
2. Combine the above with ground turkey and add chipotle chili pepper powder, smoked paprika and ground black pepper. Knead it all together and separate into four patties.
3. Cook on the grill on high heat, flipping occasionally, until desired done-ness.

Skinny Chicken Bruschetta

Prep time: 10 minutes

Cook time: 10 minutes

Serves: 4

INGREDIENTS

4 grass-fed chicken breasts

2 tomatoes

4 olives

2 onions

¼ tsp ground black pepper

1 cup roasted red pepper

3 tbsp extra virgin olive oil

INSTRUCTIONS

1. Dice the tomatoes, chop the olives and onions, and combine them with ground black pepper and 2 tbsp olive oil in a bowl and mix well into a bruschetta. Puree the roasted red pepper in a blender and set aside.
2. Combine the chicken with 1 tbsp extra virgin olive oil and cook in a pan over medium-high heat for 4 minutes, turn once, and cook another 4-6 minutes, removing from heat while still tender.
3. Place one piece of chicken on each plate and pour the roasted red pepper over each, adding bruschetta over the top. Garnish with basil and serve.

Herb Roasted Pork Tenderloin

Prep Time: 10 minutes*

Cook Time: 15 minutes

Servings: 4

INGREDIENTS

1 pork tenderloin

1 teaspoon dried rosemary

1 teaspoon dried thyme

1 teaspoon dried oregano

1 teaspoon dried basil

1 teaspoon dried marjoram (optional)

1/2 teaspoon ground black pepper

1 teaspoon Celtic sea salt

Apricot Sauce

1 cup dried apricots

2/3 cup water

1 teaspoon apple cider vinegar (or dry white wine)

INSTRUCTIONS

1. Preheat oven to 425 degrees F. Heat small pan over medium heat.
2. Rub tenderloin with salt and spices, then press into meat so it adheres. Place on sheet pan, or wire rack over sheet pan.
3. Roast for 10 - 15 minutes, until just cooked through and no pink remains. Remove pork from oven and let rest 10 minutes.

4. For *Apricot Sauce*, add dried apricots, water and vinegar to food processor or high-speed blender. Process until smooth, about 1 - 2 minutes.

5. Add *Apricot Sauce* to hot pan and reduce until slightly thickened. Stir well and do not let burn. Remove from heat.

6. Slice pork and transfer to serving dish. Top pork with *Apricot Sauce* and serve warm.

Ground Beef Stuffed Peppers

Prep Time: 10 minutes

Cook Time: 50 minutes

Servings: 4

INGREDIENTS

4 bell peppers

16 oz (1 lb) ground meat (beef, pork, chicken, turkey, etc.)

1/2 head cauliflower (1 cup riced)

1/2 cup roasted red peppers

1/4 cup sundried tomatoes

1/4 cup pecans

1/2 small onion (white, yellow or red)

2 tablespoons coconut oil

2 garlic cloves

Medium bunch fresh herbs (parsley, oregano, thyme, etc.)

1/4 teaspoon red pepper flakes

1 teaspoon ground white pepper (or black pepper)

1 teaspoon Celtic sea salt

Water

INSTRUCTIONS

1. Preheat oven to 350 degrees F.
2. Cut tops off peppers, then remove stems from tops and seeds and veins from bottoms of peppers. Leave bottoms of peppers hollow

but do not pierce. Place in baking dish just large enough to fit peppers snuggly. Set aside.

3. Peel onion and garlic. Roughly chop onions, garlic and cauliflower. Add to food processor or high-speed blender with pecans. Pulse about 15 seconds.

4. Add tops of peppers, roasted red peppers, sundried tomatoes, ground meat, salt, pepper, and fresh herbs to processor. Process until coarsely ground, about 1 - 2 minutes.

5. Use large spoon to stuff peppers with mixture. Add 1/2 cup water to bottom of baking dish. Cover peppers with aluminum foil.

6. Bake 30 minutes. Carefully remove foil and continue baking uncovered 10 - 20 minutes, until stuffing is golden brown and cooked through .

7. Carefully remove from oven and transfer peppers to serving dish. Serve hot.

Stuffed Cabbage in Tomato Sauce

Prep Time: 15 minutes

Cook Time: 60 minutes

Servings: 6

INGREDIENTS

1 large cabbage head

Filling

2 1/2 lbs ground beef

4 cage-free eggs

1/2 onion (yellow or white)

1/3 cup almond flour

1/2 cup cauliflower (riced or minced)

1/2 teaspoon dried thyme

1/2 teaspoon ground black pepper (or ground white pepper)

1 1/2 teaspoons Celtic sea salt

Tomato Sauce

2 cans (15 oz) organic tomato sauce

1/2 cup golden raisins

1/2 onion (yellow or white)

2 tablespoons raw honey (or agave or date butter)

2 tablespoons apple cider vinegar

1 1/2 teaspoons Celtic sea salt

1 teaspoon ground black pepper (or ground white pepper)

2 tablespoons bacon fat (or coconut oil or ghee)

INSTRUCTIONS

1. Preheat oven to 350 degrees F. Bring large pot of salted water to boil.

2. Carefully place cabbage head in boiling water for about 5 minutes. Use tongs to peel each layer of leaves from head as soon as they become tender. Set leaves aside on sheet pan to cool.

3. For *Tomato Sauce*, peel and mince onions. Add 1/2 of onions to medium mixing bowl. Add tomato sauce, honey, vinegar, raisins, salt and spices and mix to combine.

4. For *Filling*, add remaining onions to large mixing bowl. Mince or rice cauliflower and add to bowl with eggs, almond flour, salt, spices, and 1 cup *Tomato Sauce*. Mix well with hands or large wooden spoon.

5. Cut hard rib from bottom of each cooled cabbage leaf. Place 1/3 - 1/2 cup *Filling* near the bottom edge of cabbage leaf and roll into a neat package, tucking in sides as you roll. Repeat with remaining filling and cabbage.

6. Spread 1 cup *Tomato sauce* along bottom of deep, lidded baking dish. Place 1/2 the cabbage rolls in baking dish. Add 1/2 remaining sauce, the remaining cabbage rolls. Top with remaining sauce.

7. Tightly cover dish with lid and bake for 1 hour, until meat is cooked through and veggies are tender.

8. Transfer to serving dish and serve hot.

Slow Cooker Beef Pot Roast

Prep Time: 20 minutes

Cook Time: 6 hours

Servings: 8

INGREDIENTS

5 lb bone-in beef pot roast (or bone-in beef chuck)

2 1/2 cups chicken stock (or broth)

1 1/2 cups button mushrooms (about 1/2 pint)

3 carrots

2 celery stalks

1 onion (white or yellow)

2 garlic cloves

2 1/2 tablespoons tapioca flour (or arrowroot powder)

1 tablespoon organic tomato paste

2 sprigs fresh thyme

1 sprig fresh rosemary

1 - 2 tablespoons ground black pepper

1 - 2 tablespoons Celtic sea salt

1 tablespoon ghee (or cacao butter)

2 tablespoons coconut oil (for cooking)

INSTRUCTIONS

1. Heat large skillet over medium-high heat. Add coconut oil to hot pan.

2. Generously season beef on all sides with salt and pepper. Sprinkle 1 tablespoon tapioca or arrowroot over beef and pat to coat. Add to hot oiled pan and sear on all sides until browned, about 5 minutes per side. Set aside in baking dish to rest.

3. Slice mushrooms. Peel and chop onions. Peel and mince garlic.

4. Add ghee or butter and mushrooms to hot pan. Sauté about 2 minutes.

5. Add onions and sauté until translucent, about 5 minutes. Add garlic and sauté about 1 minute.

6. Stir in remaining 1 1/2 tablespoons tapioca or arrowroot and cook about 1 minute. Stir in tomato paste.

7. Slowly stir in chicken stock and bring to simmer, about 5 minutes. Remove from heat.

8. Roughly chop carrots and celery. Add to bottom of slow cooker. Place rested beef over veggies and pour in any juices from beef. Add rosemary and thyme. Add mushroom mixture over beef.

9. Cover slow cooker with lid. Turn on to high and cook 5 - 6 hours, until beef is fork tender.

10. Turn off slow cooker and carefully remove lid. Skim off any fat from surface and remove bones.

11. Transfer to serving dish and serve hot.

Slow Cooker Beef Burgundy

Prep Time: 30 minutes

Cook Time: 7 hours

Servings: 6

INGREDIENTS

3 lbs boneless stew beef

2 cups beef stock (or broth)

1 bottle (750 ml) organic dry red wine

1/2 cup organic sparkling apple cider (or cognac)

8 oz (1/2 lb) nitrate-free bacon

1 pint fresh mushrooms (about 2 cups)

4 large carrots

2 yellow onions

2 cups whole pearl onions (peeled)

2 garlic cloves

1 tablespoon organic tomato paste

3 tablespoons tapioca flour (arrowroot powder)

1/2 teaspoon dried thyme

1 teaspoon ground black pepper

2 teaspoons Celtic sea salt

2 tablespoons coconut oil (for cooking)

INSTRUCTIONS

1. Heat large skillet over medium-high heat. Add coconut oil to hot pan.

2. Cut beef into chunks than add to large mixing bowl. Season beef with salt and pepper, then add 2 tablespoons tapioca or arrowroot. Toss to coat.

3. Add seasoned beef to hot oiled pan in batches to brown, about 5 minutes per batch. Set aside in slow cooker.

4. Chop bacon and add to hot pan. Sauté until just crisp and fat renders out, about 5 - 8 minutes. Set aside in slow cooker.

5. Peel and chop yellow onions. Peel and mince garlic. Add to hot bacon grease and sauté about 5 minutes. Set aside in slow cooker.

6. Cut mushrooms in half. Add to hot pan with tomato paste, remaining tapioca or arrow root, thyme and apple cider. Stir to combine. Then add beef stock to deglaze pan. Bring to simmer, about 5 minutes.

7. Pour mushroom mixture into slow cooker. Add red wine and peeled pearl onions. Chop carrots and add to slow cooker. Stir to combine.

8. Cover slow cooker with lid. Turn on to low and cook 6 - 8 hours, until meat and veggies are tender.

9. Turn off slow cooker and carefully remove lid.

10. Transfer to serving dish and serve hot.

Spicy Thai Soup

Prep Time: 15 minutes

Cook Time: 1 hour

Servings: 4

INGREDIENTS

1 3/4 lbs boneless skinless chicken thighs

4 cups chicken broth (or stock)

1 can (14 oz) coconut milk (lite or full-fat)

1 1/2 cups white mushrooms

2 lemongrass stalks

1 small red onion

3 garlic cloves

3 inch piece ginger root

2 tablespoons pure fish sauce

1 1/2 teaspoons red curry paste

2 limes

1 jalapeño pepper

Small bunch cilantro

1 tablespoon coconut oil

Water

INSTRUCTIONS

1. Thinly slice bottom 2/3 of lemongrass. Peel chop garlic and ginger. Add to medium pot with chicken broth. Heat over medium-high-heat and bring to boil.

2. Reduce heat to low and simmer for 30 minutes. Strain liquid and reserve.

3. Heat pot over medium heat. Add coconut oil to hot pot.

4. Roughly chop chicken and add to hot oiled pot. Sauté and brown for 5 minutes. Quarter mushrooms and add to pot. Sauté for 5 minutes.

5. Stir in red curry paste, fish sauce, and juice of 1 lime. Add reserved chicken broth and coconut milk. Stir to combine and bring to a simmer.

6. Reduce heat to low and simmer 15 - 20 minutes. Skim off and discard any excess fat that rises to the top.

7. Peel and slice red onion. Add to pot and stir. Cook about 5 minutes, until onion softens.

8. Remove from heat. Roughly chop add 1/2 to pot and stir to combine.

9. Slice jalapeño into rings and cut lime into wedges.

10. Transfer to serving dish. Sprinkle remaining cilantro and jalapeño slices over dish.

11. Serve hot with lime wedges.

Sweet Potato & Bacon Soup

Prep Time: 20 minutes

Cook Time: 1 hour 20 minutes

Servings: 4

INGREDIENTS

4 cups chicken broth (or veggie broth)

2 large sweet potatoes (yams)

8 oz (1/2 lb) nitrate free bacon

1 cup full-fat coconut milk

1/4 teaspoon cayenne pepper

1/2 teaspoon ground cinnamon

1/2 teaspoon dried thyme

1 teaspoon ground black pepper

Celtic sea salt, to taste

INSTRUCTIONS

1. Preheat oven to 400 degrees F. Line sheet pan with parchment or baking mat.

2. Cut sweet potatoes crosswise into thick slices and lay on prepared sheet pan. Sprinkle with salt and pepper, to taste.

3. Roast sweet potatoes for about 45 minutes, until golden brown and cooked through. Remove from oven and allow to cool slightly. Then remove skin from sweet potatoes.

4. Heat medium pot over medium-high heat.

5. Chop bacon and add to hot pot. Sauté bacon until crisp, about 7 - 8 minutes. Remove bacon and set aside.

6. Add bacon fat to food processor or high-speed blender with peeled sweet potatoes and broth. Process until puréed.

7. Or add peeled sweet potatoes and broth to pot and purée in with immersion blender.

8. Add spices and coconut milk and stir to combine. Reduce heat to medium and let simmer about 10 minutes.

9. Transfer to serving dish and sprinkle with crisp bacon. Serve hot.

Parchment Baked Salmon

Prep Time: 5 minutes

Cook Time: 20 minutes

Servings: 1

INGREDIENTS

8 oz salmon fillet (deboned, skin-on)

6 - 8 medium asparagus stalks

1/2 lemon

1 basil sprig

1 rosemary sprig

1 teaspoon coconut oil

Pinch black pepper

Pinch sea salt

Parchment paper

Kitchen twine

INSTRUCTIONS

1. Place large sheet pan on bottom rack of oven. Preheat oven to 400 degrees F. prepare parchment sheet.

2. Place salmon in middle of parchment sheet skin-side down and sprinkle with salt and pepper. Place asparagus stalks next to salmon. Cut lemon into thin slices and place over fish and asparagus. Rub herbs between palms, then lay basil and rosemary sprig over lemon slices. Drizzle 1 teaspoon coconut oil over salmon and asparagus.

3. Gather edges of parchment up over salmon and tie tightly with kitchen twine to form sealed pouch.

4. Place pouch directly on hot baking sheet in hot oven. Bake for 20 minutes.

5. Remove from oven and carefully transfer pouch to serving plate. Carefully open pouch to release steam.

6. Serve hot.

Chicken Fries with Garlic Aioli

Prep Time: 10 minutes

Cook Time: 15 minutes

Servings: 2

INGREDIENTS

8 oz boneless, skinless chicken breast

1 egg

1/2 cup almond meal

1 teaspoon flax meal (or ground chia seed)

1 teaspoon ground black pepper

1/2 teaspoon paprika

1/2 teaspoon onion powder

1/2 teaspoon garlic powder

1/2 teaspoon chili powder

1/2 teaspoon sea salt

Garlic Aioli

1/2 - 3/4 cup coconut oil

1 egg yolk

2 garlic cloves

1/2 small lemon

1/4 teaspoon ground white pepper (or black pepper)

1/4 teaspoon sea salt

3 tablespoons flavorful oil (black truffle, walnut, almond, sesame, etc.)

(optional)

INSTRUCTIONS

1. Heat large pan over medium-high heat and coat with coconut oil.

2. For *Garlic Aioli*, peel garlic and add to food processor or blender with egg yolk, juice of 1/2 lemon, salt and pepper. Process until smooth, scraping down sides of vessel.

3. While processor or blender is running, very slowly drizzle in enough coconut oil to create thick mayo-like mixture. Drizzle in flavorful oil as well will processor runs (optional). If mixture is runny, drizzle in more coconut oil while processor runs until thickened. Pour into serving dish and refrigerate.

4. Slice chicken into half width-wise, creating twice the fillets. Try to slice at thickest portion to keep all fillets equal thickness.

5. Slice chicken fillets into long, 1/2 inch wide strips. Place strips between two paper towels and press to absorb excess moisture.

6. In a shallow dish, blend almond meal, flax or chia meal, spices and salt.

7. Beat egg in small mixing bowl. Toss chicken strips in beaten egg to lightly coat, then dredge in seasoned almond meal.

8. Carefully place coated chicken strips into hot oil and fry about 2 - 3 minutes, until golden brown and cooked through. Turn with tongs half way through cooking.

9. Drain cooked chicken on paper towel, then transfer to serving dish.

10. Serve hot with *Garlic Aioli*.

Ethiopian Beef Stew

Prep Time: 30 minutes

Cook Time: 1 hour

Servings: 4

INGREDIENTS

24 oz (1 1/2 lb) stew beef

2 cups beef stock (or chicken or veggie stock)

2 tablespoons organic tomato paste

1/2 teaspoon raw honey (or agave or date butter)

1 small onion

2 garlic cloves

2 teaspoons Celtic sea salt

2 teaspoons *Spice Blend*

2 tablespoons ghee (or cacao butter or bacon fat)

3 tablespoons coconut oil (or bacon fat)

Spice Blend

1/8 teaspoon ground nutmeg

1/8 teaspoon ground allspice

1/8 teaspoon turmeric

1/4 teaspoon ground cumin

1/4 teaspoon ground cinnamon

1/4 teaspoon ground cloves

1/4 teaspoon garlic powder

1/2 teaspoon ground black pepper

1/2 teaspoon ground fenugreek

1/2 teaspoon ground ginger

1/2 teaspoon ground coriander

1/2 teaspoon cardamom seed (or 1/4 teaspoon ground cardamom)

1 teaspoon dried onion flakes (or 1/2 teaspoon onion powder)

1 tablespoon paprika

2 tablespoons red pepper flakes

INSTRUCTIONS

1. Heat medium pot over medium-high heat. Add Spice blend and toast until fragrant. Stir frequently and do not burn. Remove toasted *Spice Blend* and set aside.
2. Add ghee and coconut oil to hot pot.
3. Cut beef into 1 inch chunks. Set aside.
4. Peel onion and garlic. Mince garlic and dice onion. Add to hot oiled pot and sauté until caramelized, about 2 - 3 minutes.
5. Add tomato paste, 2 teaspoons *Spice Blend* and honey to pot. Stir and cook into thick paste, about 2 minutes. Stir in a few tablespoon of beef stock to loosen paste.
6. Add beef, remaining beef stock and salt to pot. Stir to combine. Reduce heat to medium-low and simmer until beef is tender and sauce thickens and reduces, about 1 hour. Stir occasionally.
7. Transfer to serving dish and serve room temperature.

Veggie Musakhan

Prep time: 4 minutes

Cook time: 8 minutes

Servings: 4

INGREDIENTS

4 pieces grass-fed chicken thighs

1 onion

2 cloves garlic

3/4 cup sliced carrots

2 handfuls Kale greens

2 tbsp chinese five spice

2 tbsp smoked paprika

2 tbsp chipotle chili pepper powder

1 tbsp olive oil

2 tsp lemon juice

1 tbsp coconut oil

INSTRUCTIONS

1. Mince garlic and chop onion to desired size (medium strips work best). Chop carrots to 1/4" thickness. De-rib the kale and chop it coarsely, wash it and allow water to remain on the leaves. Bring 4 cups of water to a light boil.

2. Heat 1 tbsp olive oil over medium heat in a large pan. Add carrot and onion and cook for 8 minutes, stirring occasionally.

3. Meanwhile, heat 1 tbsp coconut oil over medium heat in a separate pan. Add chicken and cook for 4 minutes. Season chicken with chinese five spice, chipotle chili pepper powder and smoked paprika and turn, adding more of each spice to the other side of the chicken, cooking for another 4 minutes or until cooked through.

4. Add kale to boiling water and boil until bright green, about 5 minutes. Remove from water and let sit while the vegetables and chicken continue cooking.

5. Add everything into the pan with the vegetables and add 2 tsp lemon juice. Add minced garlic and stir for 1 minute.

6. Serve immediately.

Braised Lamb in Tomato Sauce

Prep Time: 20 minutes

Cook Time: 9 hours

Servings: 4

INGREDIENTS

3 lbs bone-in lamb shank

1 can (15 oz) organic tomato sauce

1 can (15 oz) organic crushed tomatoes

1/4 cup red wine (or apple cider vinegar)

2 cups pearl onions (peeled)

2 garlic cloves

1 teaspoon dried oregano

1 teaspoon dried thyme

1 teaspoon paprika

1 teaspoon ground black pepper

2 teaspoons Celtic sea salt

1 tablespoon coconut oil (for cooking)

Chicken stock (or water)

INSTRUCTIONS

1. Heat medium skillet over medium-high heat. Add coconut oil to hot pan.

2. Add lamb to hot oiled pan and sear on all sides, about 3 - 4 minutes per side. Set aside in slow cooker.

3. Peel pearl onions. Peel and mince garlic. Add to hot oiled pan and sauté about 2 minutes.

4. Add tomatoes sauce, red wine or vinegar, salt and spices to pan. Stir to combine.

5. Add to slow cooker with crushed tomatoes enough chicken stock or water to cover lamb.

6. Cover slow cooker with lid. Turn on to medium and cook 4 - 5 hours, until meat is tender.

7. Turn off slow cooker and carefully remove lid.

8. Transfer to serving dish and serve hot.

Garlic Sesame Chicken

Prep Time: 10 minutes

Cook Time: 20 minutes

Servings: 2

INGREDIENTS

12 oz (3/4 lb) boneless skinless chicken

1/4 cup almond flour

1/4 cup arrowroot powder

1 large cage-free egg white

2 teaspoon sesame seeds

1/4 teaspoon cayenne pepper

1/2 teaspoon garlic powder

1/2 teaspoon ground black pepper

1/2 teaspoon Celtic sea salt

Coconut oil (for cooking)

Garlic Sauce

1/2 yellow onion

1/2 lemon

6 garlic cloves

1/4 inch piece fresh ginger

1/4 cup date butter (or raw honey or agave)

2 tablespoons pure fish sauce

2 tablespoons coconut aminos (or tamar or liquid aminos)

2 tablespoons tamari (or liquid aminos or coconut aminos)

1/4 teaspoon ground black pepper

Water

INSTRUCTIONS

1. For *Garlic Sauce*, peel onions, garlic and ginger. Roughly chop and add to food processor or high-speed blender. Add date butter, fish sauce, coconut aminos, tamari and black pepper. Process until smooth.

2. Add sesame seeds to small pot. Heat over medium heat and toast about 2 minutes. Stir constantly. Transfer to small bowl and set aside.

3. Pour *Garlic Sauce* into pot and cook until onions and date butter until caramelized and garlic is fragrant, about 5 minutes. Stir frequently.

4. Add enough water to create saucy consistency. Stir frequently and bring to simmer. Simmer until *Garlic Sauce* is reduced by half and browned, about 5 minutes. Remove from heat and set aside.

5. Heat medium pan over medium-high heat. Coat pan with about 1/4 inch coconut oil.

6. In a shallow dish, blend almond meal, arrowroot powder, salt and spices.

7. Beat egg whites in small mixing bowl with hand mixer or whisk until light and frothy, about 2 - 4 minutes.

8. Cut chicken into 1 inch pieces. Dip chicken in egg whites, then dredge in seasoned flour mixture.

9. Carefully place coated chicken pieces into hot oil and fry about 2 - 3 minutes, until golden brown and cooked through. Turn with tongs halfway through cooking.

10. Drain cooked chicken on paper towel, then transfer to medium mixing bowl. Pour *Garlic Sauce* and 1 teaspoon toasted sesame seeds over chicken and toss to coat. Transfer to serving dish.
11. Sprinkle remaining toasted sesame seeds over dish. Serve hot.

Stewed Chicken and Dumplings

Prep Time: 10 minutes

Cook Time: 1 hour 20 minutes

Servings: 4

INGREDIENTS

2 lb whole chicken (innards removed)

6 - 10 cups water

3 carrots

3 celery stalks

1 small white onion (or yellow onion)

4 bay leaves

1 1/2 tablespoons dried thyme (or 4 sprigs fresh thyme)

1/2 teaspoon dried oregano

1 teaspoon paprika

2 teaspoon ground black pepper

1 tablespoon Celtic sea salt

Dumplings

3 cups almond flour

1/2 cup arrowroot powder

2 cage-free egg

1/2 cup coconut oil, chilled (or coconut or cacao butter, room temperature)

1/2 teaspoon baking soda

1/4 teaspoon ground bay leaf

1 teaspoon dried thyme

1/2 teaspoon ground white pepper (or ground black pepper)

1 teaspoon Celtic sea salt

Nut milk (or chicken broth or stock)

INSTRUCTIONS

1. Heat large pot over medium-high heat. Place chicken breast-down in hot pot. Sear chicken and turn to brown and render out fat for about 15 minutes.

2. Chop carrots and celery. Peel onion and mince. Add to chicken with salt and spices. Sauté about 2 minutes.

3. Add enough water to pot to cover chicken. Increase heat to high and bring to a boil. Reduce heat to medium and simmer about 30 minutes. Place lid loosely over pot to prevent splatter, if necessary.

4. For *Dumplings*, sift almond flour and arrowroot into medium mixing bowl. Cut in solid oil or butter with fork until crumbly mixture forms. Add egg, salt and spices, baking soda, and enough nut milk or chicken broth from pot to bring together soft, slightly sticky dough.

5. Carefully remove chicken from pot with long utensil and set aside. Use utensils to remove skin from chicken. Carve chicken into desired pieces and place back in back.

6. Use spoon or scoop to gently drop dough into pot. Cover with well-fitting lid and let simmer about 15 - 20 minutes, until *Dumplings* and chicken are cooked through. Gently stir soup to periodically prevent *Dumplings* from sticking. Turn over any *Dumplings* that are not submerged.

7. Remove from heat and transfer to serving dish. Serve hot.

Slim 'n' Trim Oven-Fried Chicken

Prep Time: 10 minutes

Cook Time: 60 minutes

Servings: 4

INGREDIENTS

32 oz (2 lb) bone-in, skinless chicken

3/4 cup fine almond flour

3/4 cup coarse almond meal (or almond flour)

2 cage free eggs

1/3 cup nut milk

1/2 teaspoon cayenne pepper

1 teaspoon ground black pepper

1 1/2 teaspoons paprika

1 1/2 tablespoons Celtic sea salt

Coconut oil (in spray bottle)

INSTRUCTIONS

1. Preheat oven to 350 degrees F. Fill spray bottle with warm coconut oil.

2. Line sheet pan with aluminum foil. Place metal cooling or baking rack over lined sheet pan. Generously spray metal rack with coconut oil to coat. Set second sheet pan aside.

3. Add almond meal and/or flour to small mixing bowl with 1 tablespoon salt and spices. Mix to combine with fork or whisk to break up clumps.

4. In shallow dish, beat eggs and nut milk until combined.

5. Use serving spoon or measuring cup to dust second sheet pan with layer of almond flour mixture onto. Sprinkle chicken with 1/2 tablespoon salt.

6. Dip and coat all chicken pieces in egg mixture then lay on second sheet pan, over layer of almond flour mixture. Use spoon or measuring cut to sprinkle almond flour mixture from mixing bowl over dipped chicken. Pat almond flour mixture into chicken on all sides until well coated.

7. Transfer coasted chicken to prepared wire rack. Generously spray coated chicken with coconut oil.

8. Bake 60 - 70 minutes, until coating is crisp and chicken is cooked through. Remove from oven and allow to cool at least 10 minutes. Then place crispy chicken on paper towels to drain, if desired.

9. Transfer to serving dish and serve immediately.

Southern Liver and Onions

Prep Time: 20 minutes*

Cook Time: 25 minutes

Servings: 4

INSTRUCTIONS

20 oz (1 1/4 lb) calves liver

2 onions (yellow or white)

4 slices nitrate-free bacon

1 lemon

2 tablespoons arrowroot powder

1/2 teaspoon Celtic sea salt

1/2 teaspoon cracked black pepper (or ground black pepper)

 Bacon fat or coconut oil (for cooking)

INSTRUCTIONS
1. *Remove thin outer membrane from liver and slice into 1/4 inch fillets. Add to glass container. Juice lemon into container and toss to coat. Cover well and refrigerate overnight.
2. Heat large cast-iron pan or skillet set over medium heat.
3. Cut bacon lengthwise into long, thin strips. Then cut in thirds crosswise and add to hot pan. Sauté bacon and let crisp, about 5 minutes. Stir occasionally. Decrease heat to medium-low.
4. Peel and thinly slice onions. Add to bacon and sauté until caramelized, about 10 minutes. Stir occasionally. Remove caramelized onions and bacon from pan and set aside.

5. Drain liver fillets in colander in sink. Rinse under running water, then pat dry.

6. In shallow dish, add arrowroot powder, salt and pepper. Mix with fork to combine.

7. Dredge liver slices in arrowroot mixture and shake off excess. Place coated liver fillets on a plate and coat remaining liver fillets.

8. Add 2 tablespoons bacon fat or coconut oil to hot pan. Add single layer of coated liver to hot oiled pan and sear for 1 minute per side. Place liver on paper towel to drain. Repeat with remaining liver.

9. Transfer liver to serving dish. Top with caramelized onions and bacon. Serve immediately .

Spicy Oregano Cubes

Prep time: 1 hr 10 minutes

Cook time: 16-20 minutes

Serves: 4

INGREDIENTS

1 boneless leg of lamb

5 tbsp extra virgin olive oil

2 tsp dried oregano

1 tbsp fresh parsley

1 lemon

½ eggplant

4 small onions

2 tomatoes

5 fresh bay leaves

¼ tsp Celtic sea salt

¼ tsp ground black pepper

INSTRUCTIONS

1. Cube the lamb, chop the fresh parsley, juice the lemon, slice and quarter the eggplant into thick pieces, halve the onions and quarter the tomatoes.
2. Place lamb in a bowl. Mix olive oil, oregano, parsley, lemon juice and Celtic sea salt and ground black pepper. Pour this over the lamb and mix well. Cover and marinate for 1 hour.

3. Preheat the grill. Thread the marinated lamb, eggplant, onions, tomatoes and bay leaves in evenly on each of four skewers.

4. Place the kebabs on a grill inside a grill pan and brush them evenly with the leftover marinade until the marinade is all gone. Cook over medium heat turning once the kebabs once, for about 8-10 minutes on each side, basting them whenever enough juice collects in the bottom of the grill pan.

5. Serve immediately or chill 20 minutes and then serve.

French Country Coq Au Vin

Prep Time: 30 minutes

Cook Time: 7 hours

Servings: 6

1 (5 - 7 lb) stewing chicken (innards removed)

2 cups chicken stock (or broth)

2 bottles(750 ml) organic red wine

6 oz nitrate-free bacon

2 cups button mushrooms

1 medium onion (yellow or white)

2 celery stalks

2 carrots

2 cups pearl onions (peeled)

3 garlic cloves

2 tablespoons organic tomato paste

1/4 cup tapioca flour (arrowroot powder)

6 sprigs fresh thyme

1 bay leaf

1 teaspoon ground black pepper

2 teaspoons Celtic sea salt

2 tablespoons coconut oil (for cooking)

INSTRUCTIONS

1. Heat large skillet over medium-high heat. Add coconut oil to hot pan.

2. Chop or cube bacon and add to hot pan. Sauté until just crisp and fat renders out, about 5 - 8 minutes. Set aside in slow cooker.

3. Cut chicken into on-the-bone serving pieces (legs, wings, thighs, breasts). Then add to large mixing bowl. Season chicken with salt and pepper, then add tapioca or arrowroot. Toss to coat.

4. Shake off excess flour and add seasoned chicken to hot greased pan in batches to brown, about 4 minutes per side. Set aside in slow cooker.

5. Peel and quarter yellow or white onion. Peel and smash garlic. Quarter mushrooms. Add to hot pan and sauté about 5 minutes. Set aside in slow cooker.

6. Cut carrots and celery into quarters. Add to hot pan with peeled pearl onions, tomato paste, remaining tapioca or arrowroot, and chicken stock. Stir to combine and deglaze pan. Bring to simmer, about 5 minutes.

7. Pour mixture into slow cooker. Add red wine, bay leaf and fresh thyme. Stir to combine.

8. Cover slow cooker with lid. Turn on to low and cook 6 - 8 hours, until meat and veggies are tender.

9. Turn off slow cooker and carefully remove lid. Remove celery, carrot, thyme and bay leaf.

10. Transfer to serving dish and serve hot.

Uptown Clam Chowder

Prep Time: 10 minutes

Cook Time: 1 hour 15 minutes

Servings: 4

INGREDIENTS

24 - 36 medium live littleneck clams (or other clam varieties)

2 cans (11.5) organic tomato juice (or about 6 large tomatoes)

2 cans (14.5 oz) organic crushed tomatoes

2 medium carrots

2 medium celery stalks

2 medium parsnips

1 red bell pepper

1 tablespoon tamari (or coconut aminos or liquid aminos)

1 bay leaf

1/4 teaspoon cayenne pepper

1/2 teaspoon onion powder

1 tablespoon dried oregano

1 tablespoon dried basil

1 teaspoon dried thyme

1 teaspoon ground black pepper

Celtic sea salt, to taste

1 cup clam juice (or veggie or chicken stock, or water) (optional)

INSTRUCTIONS

1. Have fishmonger shuck clams. Or carefully shuck clams yourself. Reserve clam juice. Set aside in refrigerator.

2. Juice tomatoes, if using. Add tomato juice and crushed tomatoes to medium pot. Heat pot over high heat.

3. Remove seeds, stems and veins from bell pepper. Dice bell pepper, carrot, celery, and parsnips. Add to pot with spices and salt, to taste.

4. Bring pot to boil, then reduce heat to low. Place lid loosely over pot to prevent splatter. Simmer for 45 minutes. Stir occasionally.

5. Remove lid and stir. Add clam juice, stock or water to reach desired consistency (optional).

6. Remove clams from refrigerator and chop, if desired. Add clams and juice to pot. Stir to combine.

7. Replace lid and continue cooking about 20 - 30 minutes. Stir occasionally.

8. Transfer to serving dish and serve hot.

Holiday Baked Ham

Prep Time: 10 minutes

Cook Time: 5 hours

Servings: 12

INGREDIENTS

1 (12 lb) bone-in ham

1 (20 oz) can organic pineapple rings (in juice)

1/2 cup date butter (or raw honey or agave)

1/2 cup whole cloves

1/2 cup water

1 lemon

1 lime

1 orange

About 12 pitted cherries (optional)

Toothpicks (optional)

INSTRUCTIONS

1. Preheat oven to 325 degrees F.
2. Drain pineapple juice into small mixing bowl. Juice lemon, lime and orange into bowl. Add sweetener and water. Mix well.
3. Place ham in roasting pan and score rind in crosshatch (diamond) pattern with knife.
4. Press cloves into rind. Place cherries on rind and secure with toothpick. Hang pineapple rings on cherries.

5. Pour pineapple juice mixture over ham and bake uncovered 4 - 5 hours, until internal temperature reaches 160 degrees F. Baste with juices about every 30 minutes.

6. Remove ham from oven. Remove toothpicks and carve. Serve hot.